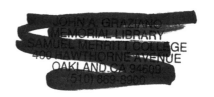

D1476896

Posterolateral Knee Injuries

Anatomy, Evaluation, and Treatment

Robert F. LaPrade, M.D., Ph.D.
Professor
Department of Orthopaedic Surgery
University of Minnesota
Minneapolis, Minnesota

Thieme
New York • Stuttgart

Thieme Medical Publishers, Inc.
333 Seventh Ave.
New York, NY 10001

Executive Editor: Esther Gumpert
Associate Editor: Owen Zurhellen IV
Vice President, Production and Electronic Publishing: Anne T. Vinnicombe
Production Editor: Print Matters, Inc.
Sales Manager: Ross Lumpkin
Chief Financial Officer: Peter van Woerden
President: Brian D. Scanlan
Compositor: Thomson Digital Services
Printer: Maple-Vail

Library of Congress Cataloging-in-Publication Data

LaPrade, Robert F.
    Posterolateral knee injuries: anatomy, evaluation, and treatment/Robert F. LaPrade.
      p.; cm.
    Includes bibliographical references and index.
    ISBN 1-58890-303-6 (US: hc.) – ISBN 3-13-140311-X (GTV:hc.)
    1. Knee–Wounds and injuries.   2. Knee–Wounds and injuries–Treatment.   I. Title. [DNLM:
    1. Knee Injuries–diagnosis.   2. Knee Injuries–history.   3. Knee Injuries–therapy.   4. Knee
    Joint–anatomy & histology. WE 870 L317p 2006]
    RD561.L34 2006
    617.5'82044–dc22

                                                                        2005046718

Important note: Medical knowledge is ever-changing. As new research and clinical experience
broaden our knowledge, changes in treatment and drug therapy may be required. The authors
and editors of the material herein have consulted sources believed to be reliable in their efforts to
provide information that is complete and in accord with the standards accepted at the time of
publication. However, in view of the possibility of human error by the authors, editors, or
publisher of the work herein or changes in medical knowledge, neither the authors, editors, or
publisher, nor any other party who has been involved in the preparation of this work, warrants
that the information contained herein is in every respect accurate or complete, and they are not
responsible for any errors or omissions or for the results obtained from use of such information.
Readers are encouraged to confirm the information contained herein with other sources. For
example, readers are advised to check the product information sheet included in the package of
each drug they plan to administer to be certain that the information contained in this publication
is accurate and that changes have not been made in the recommended dose or in the contraindications
for administration. This recommendation is of particular importance in connection with new or
infrequently used drugs.

    Some of the product names, patents, and registered designs referred to in this book are in
fact registered trademarks or proprietary names even though specific reference to this fact is not
always made in the text. Therefore, the appearance of a name without designation as proprietary
is not to be construed as a representation by the publisher that it is in the public domain.

Printed in the United States

5 4 3 2 1

TMP ISBN 1-58890-303-6
GTV ISBN 3 13 140311 X

To my wife, Sandy, and sons, Christopher, Matthew, and Jeffrey

Contents

Foreword

Posterolateral knee injuries are important for two main reasons. Grade 3 lesions do not usually heal on their own, and in combined knee injuries the posterolateral lesions are often the main problem for the patient as well as for the treating physician. Furthermore, failure to diagnose a grade 3 injury in the acute phase results in a chronic injury, which often leads to significant functional limitations during minor activities, to meniscal tears, and, if untreated, to a high incidence of arthritis over time. Similar to other areas of the body, the posterolateral anatomy of the knee has evolved through the years. Whereas our forefather-physicians Hippocrates and Galen did all their dissections in various animals, the well-known Italian anatomist and surgeon Morgagni from the University of Padova in Italy led the way in describing human anatomy and in a scientific approach to surgery. His many case studies are filled with detailed descriptions at autopsy of human anatomy, unknown to most surgeons up to that time. This book also falls into the tradition of the famous British naturalist and physician John Hunter, who practiced surgery in London at the time that the American Declaration of Independence was written in 1776. His scientific approach to dissections led to new ways of performing surgery, and he is the one who introduced the expression "clinical scientist."

With references stretching from J. B. Winslow's book in 1733 to work carried out as recently as 2003, this very first book on the posterolateral structures of the knee encompasses centuries of anatomic, biomechanical, and clinical accomplishments. It spans developments over three centuries in France, Italy, England, Germany, and Australia, in addition to the United States, and as such is written in a true international style. The author, groomed into the Hughston philosophy of anatomic restoration in human surgery, is a true clinical scientist in the best John Hunter tradition. First, he recognizes a major clinical problem through epidemiologic studies. Second, he follows the Hunter tradition with extensive dissection studies. These studies lead to trials on repair and reconstructions on cadaver specimens followed by laboratory studies on various reconstruction procedures. Then clinical studies are carried out. Thus, this book is analogous to a mystery novel with an exciting plot where the solution is found on the final page. It should stand in the current millennium as *the* book on posterolateral injuries to the knee.

Lars Engebretsen, M.D., Ph.D.
University of Oslo
Oslo, Norway

Preface

I decided to write this book because I could not find a published systematic approach to evaluating and treating posterolateral knee injuries that outlined and tied together both historical and current evaluation techniques for these injuries. In the process of writing my Ph.D. thesis on posterolateral knee injuries, I came across a wealth of information while reviewing almost all the English-language articles written on this topic. Putting together all the pieces of the puzzle allowed me to gain insight on why this area of the knee has been thought to be so difficult to understand. Because this process cannot be easily explained in brief articles or from the podium, I felt that a textbook that provides a comprehensive overview of these injuries would prove useful to medical students, residents, fellows, practicing orthopaedic surgeons, and tertiary care sports medicine specialists.

This book puts down on paper the basic principles of posterolateral knee injuries. While new information will become available in the future to help us better understand these injuries, these basic principles should be used as a basis for future understanding of these injuries and to develop a decision-making process to evaluate and treat these injuries.

The chapters are arranged to provide a progression of knowledge about posterolateral knee injuries. Although each chapter stands on its own, it is important to understand the rich body of knowledge and history behind the treatment of these injuries so one can better understand the literature. After an introductory chapter about the subject and the incidence of these injuries, the second chapter provides a comprehensive analysis of the historical literature about the anatomy and nomenclature of the posterolateral knee. Chapters 3 to 9 provide a comprehensive review of the anatomy, diagnosis, biomechanics, surgical treatment, rehabilitation, and complications. I believe that after reading this book, one should feel comfortable in dissecting posterolateral knee anatomy, clinically diagnosing posterolateral knee injuries, understanding the clinically relevant biomechanics of the posterolateral knee (and at the same time being able to apply such understanding during clinical exams), and treating injuries of the posterolateral knee.

I hope that the readers enjoy this textbook and find it to be informative and helpful in the treatment of posterolateral knee injuries. I believe they will find these injuries to be much easier to treat after reading the related chapters in this textbook.

—Robert F. LaPrade, M.D., Ph.D.

Acknowledgments

I am grateful for many things. I strongly believe that one needs to put family and faith ahead of work. At the same time, I also believe it is important not to waste a single hour that God has given us. While I am very passionate about my work, I always strive to balance the art of clinical practice, research, and teaching. I am also a father who tries to get home to be with family every night and to take the time to help with homework, to coach, or just be around my three sons.

I also recognize that one cannot be successful without surrounding oneself with good quality people. I have been very blessed in that regard at home, work, around the skating rinks and baseball diamonds, in our biomechanics lab, at church, in the classrooms and courses, and just about everywhere. I surely could not acknowledge all the great people I have been privileged to work with and encounter. There are some special people, however, who have helped to propel me into my current career path, to turn my passion about research and treating patients into this textbook.

There have been many teachers and friends who have helped push me to the point where I am now. Three high school teachers in particular deserve recognition: Ms. Kelly, Ms. Burkill, and Mrs. Jarvis. They pushed me much harder than any other teachers, and I have come to greatly appreciate the excellent work habits that they taught me.

While attending the University of Maine, I was part of an outstanding group of friends who pushed one another to achieve our best both in the classroom and in our athletic pursuits. This group includes Bill Demianiuk, Bob Stafford, Bill Berry, Jack MacDonald, Brian Donovan, Peter Cumpstone, and Charlie Wade. My cousin, Carole J. Bombard, was a wonderful cheerleader of my career choice, and later, an invaluable copyeditor of my early manuscripts. While my college professors were excellent, I remember most the advice from baseball coach John Winken: if you work a little bit every day on something you really want, you will have a good chance of achieving it.

I also appreciate the outstanding teachers I had in medical school at University of Illinois in Chicago. Two fellow medical students in particular,

Robert Swartz, M.D., and Mark Hutchinson, M.D., have been outstanding colleagues in orthopaedic surgery, and I have greatly enjoyed our journey together. I also appreciate the friendship and the hard work and support of my friends, Jeff Oken, M.D., and Mike Peters, M.D.

My residency at Michigan State University and fellowship at the Hughston Clinic in Columbus, Georgia, also provided outstanding orthopaedic training. I am grateful for the support I received from Drs. Lyne and Quinter Burnett at Michigan State in my pursuit of an academic and research career. Their support in allowing me to attend international and national meetings to present my research helped me to further define my choice of career. My appreciation and admiration of my colleagues at the Hughston Clinic is well acknowledged. Dr. Glenn Terry, Dr. Kurt Jacobson, Dr. Champ Baker, and Dr. Jack Hughston were outstanding teachers. The support of Judy Barr for her illustrations and David Curd and Cholly Minton for their research knowledge base is also much appreciated.

While I was at the University of Texas Medical Branch in Galveston, we had a great chairman, Jason Calhoun, M.D., who allowed me to pursue my desired clinical and research path. I have great appreciation for my partners, Chris Hamilton, M.D., who is now at the SCOI Clinic in Bakersfield, California, Abdul Foad, M.D., who is now an orthopaedic surgeon in Iowa, and Greg Chaljub, M.D., who provided invaluable assistance and time on our pilot MRIs for the development of protocols for these posterolateral knee injuries.

I have had many colleagues at the University of Minnesota who have also helped me to get to this point in my career. I am much indebted to Fred Wentorf, M.S., for his hard work in the lab and on many of the papers that we have published. Jack Lewis, Ph.D., has also been a steady hand in guiding the research hypothesis in the development of appropriate research protocols. Tom Gilbert, M.D., was also a driving force in the development of our MRI protocol. Liza Arendt, M.D., has been a very supportive and knowledgeable partner. And my chairman, Marc Swiontkowski, M.D., has also been very supportive of my research and has strongly encouraged me to continue my outcome studies.

While acknowledging my colleagues, I also greatly appreciate the residents and medical students who have worked with me in the lab. It has been a mutually beneficial arrangement for them to learn how to do proper research, interpret the literature, and gain a footing toward either an orthopaedic residency position or an academic career. While the list of residents and medical students who have worked in the lab is more than two pages long, several persons on the list come to mind who have pushed me a great extent in developing my own knowledge base and in turn have made it really fun to get up and go to work early in the morning or to stay late at night to finish projects. These include my first medical student at the University of Minnesota, Scott Resig, M.D., and more recently Thuan Ly, M.D., and Patrick Morgan, M.D. All of you are shining beacons for the future of orthopaedics, and it has been a pleasure to work with you.

I also have to especially acknowledge the orthopaedics biomechanic lab at the University of Minnesota, which has been a great source of basic science information that we have brought to clinical practice. I could not have accomplished all these projects without their help. Conrad Lindquist has been an invaluable team member in making devices and testing machines for our studies, and his work is truly appreciated. Andy Evanson is an excellent medical illustrator, and Nancy Eibrink works almost daily on our manuscripts and book chapters. It takes a team to get a lot of things done, and I deeply appreciate their help.

My colleagues at the University of Norway have been outstanding. Lars Engebretsen, M.D., Ph.D., had the same position that I currently have at the University of Minnesota. When he left, I took his position. We can say now that basically I was hand picked to fill his position, and I am grateful to him for that. He has been a tremendous colleague, co-worker on projects, and most importantly, a great friend. In addition, Steinar Johanson, M.D., has been an invaluable colleague on many of these projects, especially in our outcome studies. His attempts to improve my culinary education have also been appreciated.

I have not left out anybody's name intentionally in these acknowledgments, but I have tried to include those colleagues who come to mind as having most helped me to culminate my work on posterolateral knee injuries and in the publication of this book. I appreciate the help of the faculty in the Instructional Courses and Symposium, who have pushed me to continue my work and have kept inviting me back to give more lectures.

In closing, I could not have done any of this without my family and their support. My parents, grandparents, and extended family instilled in me a strong work ethic for which I am grateful. For my immediate family, I recognize how difficult it can be for me to be gone either at work, doing research, or at courses for extended periods of time. Sandy, I could not have done all this without your love and support. Your support of my career is deeply appreciated. Chris, Matt, and Jeff, my sons, you are the bright and shining points of light of my life. I consider myself the luckiest man in the world to have you as my sons.

1

Introduction and Incidence of Posterolateral Knee Injuries

Posterolateral corner knee injuries can be very problematic injuries when they are not recognized by the treating health care professional. This is especially true as the operative results of significant injuries for acute repairs are much better than chronic reconstructions. This can be compounded by the fact that we haven't as a profession developed specific diagnostic tools to help identify these injuries, and many physicians do not include the multiple varied means to clinically diagnose posterolateral corner knee injuries in their repertoire for the clinical examination of an acute or chronic ligament-injured knee. Physicians who treat acute knee injuries should heed the advice of the late Jack Hughston, M.D., with regard to the underdiagnosis of posterolateral corner knee injuries. Hughston stated on many occasions that although you may not have seen posterolateral corner knee injuries (in your practice), "I can assure you that they have seen you."

A lot of work has been performed over the last several years to facilitate the diagnosis and treatment of posterolateral knee injuries. Understanding the anatomy of the posterolateral knee has been a major problem in advancing our treatment of these injuries. For example, different treatment centers call the same structure by different names, which has made it difficult to compare studies performed by different regional or international groups, and has hindered the research progress in the treatment of these injuries. For example, we can understand the dilemma of young clinicians trying to figure out a series of podium presentations at an instructional course lecture or symposium where the presenters discuss the arcuate complex, the arcuate ligament, and the popliteofibular ligament. If these young clinicians were to read the "classic" literature, such as works by Seebacher,[1] Hughston,[2-5] or Warren's group,[6-11] they would be even more confused about the differences between these structures. In Chapter 2 I review the history of the nomenclature of the posterolateral corner of the knee over the past 250 years and try to resolve most of the confusion about these structures. In fact, quite possibly the only main structures of the posterolateral corner of the knee that have an accurate qualitative description in the literature over this time period are the fibular (lateral) collateral ligament and the popliteus tendon. There have been significant differences in the dissection techniques among many different reporting institutions over time, which has also contributed to this problem. Although it is well recognized that fresh or fresh-frozen cadaveric knee specimens are the most ideal to determine the intricate structures and arrangements of the posterolateral corner of the knee, some earlier studies used formalin-embalmed knees to report on the anatomy of the posterolateral corner of the knee. In addition, most of the studies have dissected the posterolateral corner of the knee from an outside-in approach. Although this is fairly standard for anatomists, physicians at one institution, the Hospital for Special Surgery,[7] have noted that the inside-out dissection technique helped them recognize the intricate arrangements of structures of the posterolateral corner of the knee, especially the popliteofibular ligament. In addition, one's familiarity with dissection techniques facilitates one's recognition of the arrangement of these structures and one's recognition of possibly previously undescribed fascial attachments and arrangements. I can state that in my own studies, I have significantly improved my ability to include more quantitative information in my publications over time. I believe much of this is due to experience, as well as to a large clinical practice that has helped me to recognize the important areas to look at anatomically and has helped me repair or reconstruct injuries so that patients can return to their highest level of function.

Posterolateral rotatory instability of the knee was first described in 1976 as a clinical entity that caused significant functional limitations in patients.[2] However, only in the past 10 to 15 years has the role of posterolateral knee injuries in causing abnormal knee motion become better understood. It has also become increasingly recognized that the incidence of posterolateral knee injuries and the negative effect of untreated injuries on knee function and outcome has been underreported.

The anatomy of the posterolateral knee has been recognized as being very complex, and thus the diagnosis of posterolateral knee injuries has been known to be very difficult. In evaluating acute knee injuries, there may be concurrent swelling, effusion, and generalized knee pain, which can make it difficult to recognize a posterolateral corner injury, especially if the examiner does not look for it. In addition, in the presence of other concurrent knee ligament injuries, such as of the anterior cruciate ligament, medial collateral ligament, or posterior cruciate ligament in either the acute or chronic patient, it may be difficult on physical examination to determine the neutral axis point of the knee on the anterior to posterior and medial to lateral planes,[2,10,12–15] which can make it difficult to determine on clinical examination whether there is significant injury to the posterolateral structures of the knee. In addition, it has been well recognized that the posterolateral corner of the knee has a variable amount of natural physiologic laxity among patients,[16] so it is very important to make sure that the examiner verifies that the increase of motion seen on the injured knee is compared with the natural laxity of the patient's contralateral normal knee. But when both knees are injured, it can be very difficult to discern the extent of a posterolateral injury.

Injuries to the ligaments of the knee are very common, especially in the active adolescent and young adult population. The incidence of overall complete knee ligament injuries[17] in the general population is estimated to be 1 per 1000 patients per year.[18] Of the more serious knee ligament injuries that require surgery, anterior cruciate ligament tears are the most common with about 2000 per year in Norway[19] and 100,000 per year in the United States.[20,21] It also has been estimated that the risk of an athlete tearing the anterior cruciate ligament during a competitive season is about 2%.[22] The incidence of anterior cruciate ligament tears in Norwegian Team Handball has been found to be 0.9 per 1000 player-hours, with each team having an average of one player sustaining an anterior cruciate ligament tear per year.[23,24] Only 50% of these athletes were able to return to full participation at the same level. Although the majority of reconstructions of torn anterior cruciate ligaments do well, there is still some concern that some of these reconstructions fail due to unrecognized or untreated posterolateral knee injuries.[21,25–27]

Historically, it has been reported that injuries to the posterolateral aspect of the knee occur less frequently than injuries to other knee ligaments. DeLee et al[28] noted that in the retrospective study of 735 knee ligament injuries treated in San Antonio, Texas, from 1971 through 1977, 12 patients (1.6%) had isolated acute posterolateral knee injuries, while there were 32 (4.4%) other cases of acute posterolateral knee injuries seen in association with cruciate ligament tears (total incidence, 5.8%). In Danish studies, which have looked at the incidence of knee injuries that present to an emergency room for treatment, the annual incidence of severe posterolateral knee injuries was estimated to be less than 0.1 per 1000 patients. This compared with an incidence of 0.7 for the medial collateral ligament and 0.3 for the anterior cruciate ligament per 1000 inhabitants.[18] Miller et al[29] reported a 6% incidence of posterolateral knee injuries (30 patients) in a consecutive series of 481 knee magnetic resonance imaging (MRI) scans.

However, it has been speculated[25,30] that the overall incidence of posterolateral knee injuries has been underestimated and underreported because of the difficulty in diagnosing this complex problem and because examiners do not look for it. Five studies have provided some evidence that this may be true. O'Brien et al[25] reported a 15% failure rate in a group of patients who underwent anterior cruciate ligament reconstructions, which appeared to be due to unrecognized or untreated posterolateral instability at the time of their index anterior cruciate ligament reconstruction. However, it is unclear what the total incidence of posterolateral knee injuries was in this population. Fanelli and Edson[31] reported that in a consecutive group of 222 patients with a knee hemarthrosis in a level 1 trauma center, 28.4% had posterolateral injuries. Within their group of 222 patients, 85 had posterior cruciate ligament tears, with 53 of these patients (62%) having concurrent posterolateral knee injuries along with their posterior cruciate ligament tears. In addition, with a total of 148 anterior cruciate ligament tears in this group of 222 patients, there were 18 concurrent posterolateral knee injuries in patients with anterior cruciate ligament tears (12%). Another study has reported that in a group of 100 consecutive anterior cruciate ligament reconstructions, the incidence of concurrent posterolateral instability in these knees was shown to be 11%.[30] Noyes et al[27] reported that in a consecutive series of 41 patients with anterior cruciate ligament tears, varus alignment, and varying amounts of posterolateral instability, 15 patients had a total of 19 previous anterior cruciate ligament reconstructions that had failed. They reported that many of these failures were due to unrecognized posterolateral instability.[27] Finally, another study by Noyes et al[27] reported that 18 (30%) of 57 patients who underwent a revision anterior cruciate ligament reconstruction using bone–patellar tendon–bone autografts (performed between 1990 and 1996) had untreated or unrecognized posterolateral corner injuries, which appeared to contribute to the index anterior cruciate ligament reconstruction graft failure. These studies would indicate that posterolateral knee injuries have a higher incidence than has been reported and are an important cause of cruciate ligament reconstruction graft failure.

It has been recognized in the past that the incidence of posterolateral knee injuries has been underestimated and that prospective studies were needed. In an effort to determine the incidence of posterolateral knee injuries in a prospective manner, we prospectively documented all acute knee injuries that underwent an MRI scan at the major imaging referral center in the Minneapolis–St. Paul metropolitan area. All knees that had been injured within 30 days of the scan were read by a musculoskeletal radiologist who specialized in sports medicine. We found that out of a total 331 consecutive acute knee injuries, 185 (56%) had a ligament injury. Of these 185 patients with a ligament injury, 136 patients (74%) had an anterior cruciate ligament tear, 27 (15%) had a posterior cruciate ligament tear, 72 (39%) had a medial collateral ligament tear, and 30 patients (16%) had a posterolateral corner injury. In this group of 30 patients, there were found to be 18 fibular collateral ligament tears, 17 popliteus tendon tears, and 17 popliteofibular ligament tears documented; 20 (67%) had documented posterolateral knee injuries and other concurrent ligament tears present. Overall, 9.1% of patients who presented to the imaging center for evaluation were found to have a posterolateral knee injury. Although it can be argued that MRI may not be as accurate as a good physical examination in the documentation of posterolateral corner injuries, it can also be argued that it is very difficult to obtain a large population of patients with acute knee injuries at a sports medicine referral center without some referral bias. I performed this study because I felt a large MRI study with all the acute knee injuries that presented to a major MRI referral center would provide as close as possible the actual number of posterolateral knee injuries that occur in the general population.

In summarizing the various different incidence studies that have included posterolateral knee injuries, it would appear that the incidence of posterolateral knee injuries is between 5% and 9%. Thus, it appears that the actual incidence of posterolateral knee injuries has been underestimated in the past. It is hoped that with an improved understanding of how to diagnose these complex injuries, more injuries will be recognized in the acute time frame and treated before they progress to chronic injuries.

One of the most important things to recognize about grade 3 posterolateral corner injuries is that a failure to diagnose them in the acute injury phase results in a chronic injury, which often leads to significant functional limitations during minor activities, to meniscal tears,[30] and to a high incidence of arthritis

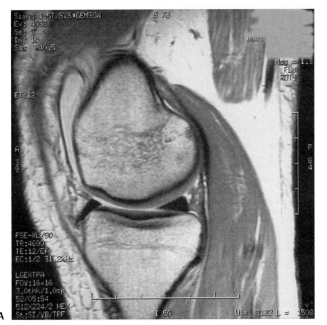 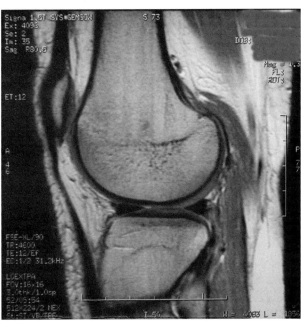

A   B

Figure 1–1   Sagittal magnetic resonance imaging (MRI) cuts of the midmedial **(A)** and midlateral **(B)** compartment of a left knee. The difference between the concave medial tibial plateau **(A)** compared with the convex bony anatomy of the lateral tibial plateau **(B)** is seen.

over time if they are not treated.[2,32–34] It has been hypothesized that untreated posterolateral corner injuries do not heal because the two opposing convex surfaces of the lateral compartment of the knee have an inherent bony instability[35,36] (**Fig. 1–1**). Unlike the medial compartment of the knee, where isolated injuries to the medial collateral ligament complex usually heal without any residual or functional laxity, in part because the concave surface of the medial tibial plateau articulates with the convex surface of the medial femoral condyle and provides an inherent amount of bony stability to the medial compartment,[37] the relatively convex surfaces of the lateral tibial plateau and lateral femoral condyle result in increased motion due to the inherent bony instability after a posterolateral corner injury, which can lead to residual knee laxity as the injured structures either do not heal or heal in a nonfunctional elongated position.[35] Also, it is well recognized that the results of an acute repair of a posterolateral corner injury are far superior to that of a chronic reconstruction.[4,28,30,38,39] With this information in mind, the examiner must be vigilant and listen to patients' description of their mechanism of injury, as well as perform a thorough clinical examination to test the integrity of all ligaments of the knee when a ligament injury is suspected, so as not to miss an acute posterolateral corner injury. The consequences to the patient of a missed acute posterolateral corner injury can be significant, due to the poorer outcomes and more extensive surgery required to treat chronic rather than acute posterolateral knee injuries.[2,4,30,38,39]

The role of combined posterolateral corner and other concurrent cruciate ligament injuries in causing significant laxity of the knee, compared with isolated cruciate ligament instability alone, has been increasingly recognized. It has been suggested that the majority of patients with posterior cruciate ligament tears and functional instability with activities have concurrent posterolateral rotatory instability of the knee that is causing their functional limitations[31,40] and that most isolated posterior cruciate ligament tears can be treated nonoperatively.[8,41,42] With this in mind, it is important to recognize the interaction and effects of posterolateral corner knee injuries on cruciate ligament reconstructions. As will be demonstrated in further chapters, concurrent repair and reconstruction of posterolateral knee injuries is required when either an anterior cruciate ligament or a posterior cruciate ligament reconstruction is performed. This is necessary to prevent increased force on these reconstruction grafts, caused by the increased motion with a posterolateral knee injury, which could ultimately contribute to the cruciate ligament graft failure.

I have undertaken this work because after 10 years of dedicated research in this particular area, I believe that many of the clinical dilemmas in treating posterolateral corner knee injuries have been resolved through my laboratory's, and other laboratories', research in this area. When I interviewed for orthopaedic sports medicine fellowships, I came to recognize that I wanted to pursue an academic sports medicine career. When I asked what were some of the most difficult problems to treat at that point in time in sports medicine, the most common problem noted was posterolateral corner knee injuries. For that reason, I chose to pursue my fellowship at the Hughston Sports Medicine Clinic so that I could learn from Glenn "Corky" Terry, M.D., as many people said he was the world's best anatomist in this area, and I was able to learn extensively from his work. I have been lucky to surround myself with research scientists who have a similar hard work ethic in order to answer many of the clinical problems that have been raised that we have seen in these patients over the last 10 years. It goes without saying that one cannot accomplish one's goals without surrounding oneself with hard-working individuals. I have been blessed in this regard.

References

1. Seebacher JR, Inglis AE, Marshall JL, Warren RF. The structure of the posterolateral aspect of the knee. J Bone Joint Surg 1982;64A:536–541
2. Hughston JC, Andrews JR, Cross MJ, Moschi A. Classification of knee ligament instabilities. Part II: the lateral compartment. J Bone Joint Surg 1976;58A:173–179
3. Hughston JC, Norwood LA. The posterolateral drawer test and external rotation recurvation test for posterolateral rotatory instability of the knee. Clin Orthop Rel Res 1980;147:82–87
4. Hughston JC, Jacobson KE. Chronic posterolateral rotatory instability of the knee. J Bone Joint Surg 1985;67A:351–359
5. Hughston JC. Knee Ligaments. Injury and Repairs. Chicago: Mosby, 1993
6. Warren LF, Marshall JL. The supporting structures of the layers on the medial side of the knee: an anatomical analysis. J Bone Joint Surg 1979;61A:56–62
7. Maynard MJ, Deng X-H, Wickiewicz TL, Warren RF. The popliteofibular ligament: rediscovery of a key element in posterolateral instability. Am J Sports Med 1996;24:311–316
8. Veltri DM, Warren RF. Isolated and combined posterior cruciate ligament injuries. J Am Acad Orthop Surg 1993;1:67–75

 9. Veltri DM, Warren RF. Anatomy, biomechanics, and physical findings in postero-lateral knee instability. Clin Sports Med 1994;13:599–614
10. Veltri DM, Deng X-H, Torzilli PA, Warren RF, Maynard MJ. The role of the cruci-ate and posterolateral ligaments in stability of the knee. Am J Sports Med 1995;23:436–443
11. Veltri DM, Deng X-H, Torzilli PA, Maynard MJ, Warren RF. The role of the popli-teofibular ligament in stability of the human knee: a biomechanical study. Am J Sports Med 1996;24:19–27
12. Grood ES, Noyes FR, Butler DL, Suntay WJ. Ligamentous and capsular restraints preventing straight medial and lateral laxity in intact human cadaver knees. J Bone Joint Surg 1981;63A:1257–1269
13. Gollehon DL, Torzilli PA, Warren RF. The role of the posterolateral and cruciate ligaments in the stability of the human knee: a biomechanical study. J Bone Joint Surg 1987;69A:233–242
14. Grood ES, Stowers SF, Noyes FR. Limits of movement in the human knee: effect of sectioning the posterior cruciate ligament and posterolateral structures. J Bone Joint Surg 1988;70A:88–97
15. Markolf KL, Wascher DC, Finerman GA. Direct *in vitro* measurement of forces in the cruciate ligaments. Part II: the effects of section of the posterolateral struc-tures. J Bone Joint Surg 1993;75A:387–394
16. Cooper DE. Tests for posterolateral instability of the knee in normal subjects. J Bone Joint Surg 1991;73A:30–36
17. American Medical Association (AMA). Standard Nomenclature of Athletic In-juries. Chicago: American Medical Association, 1966
18. Nielsen AB, Yde J. Epidemiology of acute knee injuries: a prospective hospital investigation. J Trauma 1991;31:1644–1648
19. Engebretsen L, Tegnander A, Benum P. Treatment of ACL injuries in Norway: a com-parison with the ACL study group. Tidsskr Nor Laegeforer 1989;109:1288–1290
20. Johnson DL, Harner CD, Maday MG, Fu FH. Revision anterior cruciate ligament surgery. In: Fu F, Harner CD, Vince KG, eds. Knee Surgery. Baltimore: Williams & Wilkins, 1994:877–895
21. Noyes FR, Barber-Westin SD. Revision of anterior cruciate surgery with use of bone-patellar tendon-bone autogenous grafts. J Bone Joint Surg 2001;83A: 1131–1143
22. LaPrade RF, Burnett QM II. Femoral intercondylar notch stenosis and correlation to anterior cruciate ligament injuries: a prospective study. Am J Sports Med 1994;22:198–203
23. Myklebust G, Maehlum S, Engebretsen L, Strand T, Solgheim E. Registration of cruciate ligament injuries in Norwegian top level handball. Scand J Med Sci Sports 1997;7:289–292
24. Myklebust G, Maehlum S, Holm I, Bahr R. A prospective cohort study of ACL in-juries in elite Norwegian team handball. Scand J Med Sci Sports 1998;8:149–153
25. O'Brien SJ, Warren RF, Pavlov H, Panariello R, Wickiewicz TL. Reconstruction of the chronically insufficient anterior cruciate ligament with the central third of the patellar ligament. J Bone Joint Surg 1991;73A:278–286
26. LaPrade RF, Terry GC. Injuries to the posterolateral aspect of the knee: associa-tion of anatomic injury patterns with clinical instability. Am J Sports Med 1997;25:433–438
27. Noyes FR, Barber-Westin SD, Hewitt TE. High tibial osteotomy and ligament reconstruction for varus angulated anterior cruciate ligament deficient knees. Am J Sports Med 2000;28:282–296

28. DeLee JC, Riley MB, Rockwood CA. Acute posterolateral rotatory instability of the knee. Am J Sports Med 1983;11:199–207
29. Miller TT, Gladden P, Staron RB, Henry JH, Feldman F. Posterolateral stabilizers of the knee: anatomy and injuries assessed with MR imaging. AJR Am J Roentgenol 1997;169:1641–1647
30. LaPrade RF, Hamilton CD, Engebretsen L. Treatment of acute and chronic combined anterior cruciate ligament and posterolateral knee ligament injuries. Sports Med Arth Rev 1997;5:91–99
31. Fanelli GC, Edson CJ. Posterior cruciate ligament injuries in trauma patients. Part II: arthroscopy 1995;11:526–529
32. Bousquet G, Charmion L, Passot JP, Girardin P, Relave M, Gazielly D. Stabilization du condyle externe du genou dans les laxiries anterieures chroniques. Rev Chir Orthop Reparatrice Appar Mot 1986;72:427–434
33. Kannus P. Nonoperative treatment of grade II and III sprains of the lateral ligament compartment of the knee. Am J Sports Med 1989;17:83–88
34. Stäubli HU. Posteromedial and posterolateral capsular injuries associated with posterior cruciate ligament insufficiency. Sports Med Arthro Rev 1994;2:146–164
35. Jakob RP, Hassler H, Stäubli HU. Observations on rotatory instability of the lateral compartment of the knee: experimental studies on the functional anatomy and pathomechanism of the true and reversed pivot shift sign. Acta Orthop Scand Suppl 1981;191:1–32
36. LaPrade RF. The medial collateral ligament complex and posterolateral aspect of the knee. In: Sports Medicine Orthopaedic Knowledge Update (OKU). Chicago: American Academy of Orthopaedic Surgeons, 1999
37. Indelicato PA, Hermansdorfer J, Huegel M. Nonoperative management of complex tears of the medial collateral ligament of the knee in intercollegiate football players. Clin Orthop Rel Res 1990;256:174–177
38. Baker CL, Norwood LA, Hughston JC. Acute combined posterior cruciate and posterolateral instability of the knee. Am J Sports Med 1983;11:308–314
39. Krukhaug Y, Molster A, Rodt A, Strand T. Lateral ligament injuries of the knee. Knee Surg Sports Traumatol Arthrosc 1998;6:21–25
40. Müller W. The Knee: Form, Function and Ligament Reconstruction. New York: Springer-Verlag, 1983
41. Harner CD, Höher J. Evaluation and treatment of posterior cruciate ligament injuries. Am J Sports Med 1998;26:471–482
42. Shelbourne KD, Davis TJ, Patel DV. The natural history of acute, isolated, nonoperatively treated posterior cruciate ligament injuries: a prospective study. Am J Sports Med 1999;27:276–283

2

History of the Nomenclature and Study of the Anatomy of the Posterolateral Knee

It is well recognized that the anatomy of the posterolateral corner of the knee is more complex than that on the medial side. This is partly due to the developmental phylogeny of the knee that has evolved between species over time. In lower animal species, the fibula articulates with the femur, and it has descended over eons to articulate with the tibia in higher order animal species.[1-5] Previous studies have reported that in lower animal species, there is a meniscus between the articulation of the femur and the fibular head.[1,2,4-6] Many authors have theorized that this femorofibular meniscus evolved into the popliteus tendon of the knee.[1-5] In addition to these changes that have been noted in the popliteus complex, the biceps femoris complex in other animal species has attachments around the knee that are significantly different from those found in humans.[4,6-8] It has also been reported that the human knee is the only one that has an iliotibial band over the lateral aspect of the knee.[7,9]

The bony anatomy of the lateral aspect of the knee is also an indirect contributing factor to the complexity of its anatomy. Although the medial femoral condyle, with its convex surface, and the medial tibial plateau, with its concave surface, have two opposing surfaces that are inherently stable as they cup together, one can see that this is not true for the lateral compartment of the knee. Both the lateral femoral condyle and the lateral tibial plateau have convex surfaces that make the bony geometry inherently unstable.[10,11] The two convex surfaces rely on point contact to provide bony stability to the lateral compartment of the knee. This inherently unstable bony geometry places increased reliance on the integrity of the multiple individual soft tissue structures of the posterolateral aspect of the knee to provide static stability for the lateral side of the knee (**Fig. 2–1**). In addition, when the posterolateral structures of the knee are injured, there is less ability for these structures to remain in opposition, so there is less ability for these structures to heal.

The difference in the inherent stability of the medial and lateral menisci also contributes to differences in the inherent stability and healing potential between the two tibiofemoral compartments. The medial meniscus has a more stable meniscotibial attachment and has less relative motion across the medial tibial plateau with flexion and extension of the knee. However, the lateral meniscus is much less stable and has a less restraining meniscotibial attachment, which results in far greater motion of the lateral meniscus with knee motion than its medial counterpart.[12] The increased lateral meniscal motion further accentuates the unstable bony geometry of the lateral compartment of the knee.

In addition to the confusion about posterolateral knee anatomy from its developmental phylogeny and bony anatomy differences, there has also been a great deal of confusion created by varying anatomic descriptions of these structures by anatomists and physicians studying these structures. Over the last century and a half, several published articles have described the anatomy of the posterolateral knee using varying nomenclature, descriptions, and illustrations. The variations in nomenclature used in different reporting institutions have especially contributed to the confusion regarding the anatomy of the posterolateral corner of the knee.

A careful review of the literature reveals that a lot of the confusion about the nomenclature of posterolateral knee structures may be due to the revision of the standard anatomic nomenclature by the International Congress of Anatomists late in the first half of the 20th century. Their combined efforts to update the nomenclature of the knee resulted in the *Nomina Anatomica*,[13] which attempted to modernize previous anatomic descriptions. As one author from that time pointed out,[14] however, the short external lateral ligament (which appears to be the popliteofibular ligament in his descriptions) was omitted from the nomenclature revision. As a result of this omission, this structure has not been specifically depicted or described well in anatomic textbooks since that point in time. It appears that a lot of the confusion about the nomenclature of the posterolateral knee is due to this omission, because varying authors have attempted to describe this structure in many different ways over the past 50 years. In fact, other authors who have quoted Last[14] since his publication in 1950 seem to be describing the short external lateral ligament as a different structure than what he had originally described it to be.[4,15,16] A review of these previous studies and a scholarly interpretation of which structures they may be referring to are presented on a structure-by-structure basis in this chapter in an attempt to resolve this confusion and to present the case for a descriptive anatomic nomenclature basis for the posterolateral structures presented in Chapter 3. It is important to understand that a unified nomenclature for the posterolateral knee is essential to elucidate the contributions of each structure to knee stability and joint function, and to accurately compare anatomic, biomechanical, clinical, and radiographic imaging studies.

◆ Fibular Collateral Ligament (Lateral Collateral Ligament)

In one of the early studies in the English-language literature on the anatomy of the posterolateral knee, Sutton[17] reported in 1884 on the anatomy of the "external lateral ligament of the knee joint," which we now know to be the

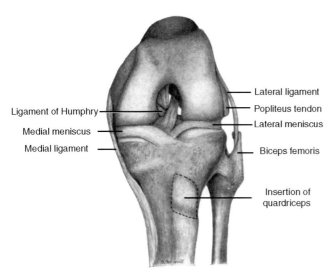

Ligament of Humphry

Medial meniscus

Medial ligament

Lateral ligament

Popliteus tendon

Lateral meniscus

Biceps femoris

Insertion of quardriceps

Figure 2–1 Lateral ligament (fibular collateral ligament) of the knee joint coursing from the lateral femoral condyle to the fibula with the biceps femoris enveloping the fibular attachment. (From Last RJ. Some anatomical details of the knee joint. J Bone Joint Surg 1948;30B:683–688, with permission.)

fibular collateral ligament. Sutton described it as extending over the lateral aspect of the knee, and he theorized that this ligament was an extension of the peroneus longus muscle and tendon to the knee. He felt that it was an extension of these structures due to his comparative anatomy studies in other animal species. These species included the opossum, domestic ox, and the gibbon.

Last[18] reported in 1948 that the lateral ligament of the knee joint of "current" British terminology was represented by the long external lateral ligament of "old terminology" (**Fig. 2–1**). He reported that it originated from the lateral epicondyle of the femur and inserted on the fibular head. Last also observed that the tendon of the biceps femoris wrapped around the posterior aspect of the lateral ligament of the knee.

In an article on the prenatal development of the human knee, Gray and Gardner[19] reported that the fibular collateral ligament was present in a 9-week-old fetus as a thin cellular band that descended from the lateral aspect of the femoral condyle to the fibular head. By 14 weeks of age in the fetus, the fibular collateral ligament resembled that of the adult knee. They reported that their findings in the fetus indicated that the fibular collateral ligament developed in situ, and that there was no evidence to support Sutton's[17] theory that the fibular collateral ligament was an extension of the peroneus longus fascia over the lateral compartment of the leg.

Kaplan[20] in 1957 reported that the most important structure found under the fascia on the lateral side of the knee was the lateral collateral ligament. He reported that this ligament coursed between the lateral condylar tubercle, which we now call the lateral epicondyle, of the femur and the middle of the lateral surface of the fibular head.

In summarizing these representative previous studies that have described the fibular collateral ligament, it appears that the course and qualitative attachment sites of the fibular collateral ligament were agreed upon by the authors of these previous studies. The fibular collateral ligament was noted to attach in the region of the lateral epicondyle on the lateral aspect of the fibular head; it coursed distally to attach to the lateral aspect of the fibular head, and was surrounded by components of the biceps femoris along its distal course.

◆ Popliteus Complex and Popliteofibular Ligament

To understand the complex anatomy of the popliteus complex, it is very important to review both older human literature and comparative anatomy studies. It is especially clear that this portion of the anatomy of the posterolateral knee has been one of the most confusing for clinicians to understand. A large part of this confusion is due to the fact that the popliteus attachment to the fibular head (the popliteofibular ligament) was omitted from much, but not all, of the English-language orthopaedic literature for much of the latter part of the 20th century. Those articles that recognized this structure were in more obscure orthopaedic or anatomy journals that went unread by most practicing orthopaedists. Therefore, many different descriptions with varying nomenclature of the structures in this area emerged over time.

Higgins[21] reported that the proximal attachments of the popliteus complex were to the lateral femoral condyle and the fibular head. The fibular attachment was noted to consist of two strong and distinct bands. In addition, Higgins noted attachment fibers from the popliteus to the posterior joint capsule, the coronary ligament to the lateral meniscus, and the lateral meniscus itself. The femoral attachment of the popliteus was noted to be in a groove on the femur and distal and anterior to the "long external lateral ligament" (fibular collateral ligament). The popliteus tendon was also noted to form a groove where it crossed the posterolateral aspect of the lateral tibial plateau. We now know that his studies described, in an accurate qualitative manner, the anterior and posterior divisions of the popliteofibular ligament, the popliteomeniscal fascicles, and the popliteal aponeurotic attachments to the lateral meniscus.

Fürst[1] reported in the German literature in 1903 that the tendon of the popliteus and its muscle were two structures that developed independently in the animal world. He reported that the popliteus muscle attached directly to the fibular head in lower animal species. These lower animal species were also noted to have a meniscus between the fibula and femur. The popliteus tendon was felt to have evolved from this femorofibular meniscus. In humans, Fürst reported that the popliteus muscle had two proximal attachments, with one on the lateral femoral condyle (the popliteus tendon attachment to the femur) and the other on the fibular head (the popliteofibular ligament). Fürst also noted that the popliteus tendon created a small sinusoidal cartilage indentation (which Stäubli and Birrer[22] noted as the sulcus statorious of Fürst) on the border of the lateral femoral condyle of the knee near full extension. Fürst felt that the sulcus statorious was acquired due to the upright posture of humans and that the popliteal sulcus on the lateral femoral condyle evolved due to the flexed knee position in gait of most lower animal species.

Taylor and Bonney[2] reported that in reptiles the popliteus muscle originated from the fibular head and also had a small attachment to the femorofibular meniscus. This femorofibular meniscus attached to the lateral femoral condyle via a femorofibular ligament. In addition, they noted that some lower animals and marsupials had a popliteus muscle that attached to the fibular head. However, in higher marsupial species such as kangaroos, and in most higher mammals, the popliteus acquired its femoral attachment by the development of the femorofibular meniscus, and its femorofibular ligamentum attachment, to evolve to form the popliteus tendon femoral attachment. The authors also noted that in higher mammals, in which motion between the tibia and fibula were more important, the popliteus attained a firm attachment to the fibular head. We now know that this structure is the popliteofibular ligament.

Haines[6] also performed extensive comparative anatomy studies of the posterolateral aspect of the knee. He reported that in the crocodile, which appears to have the most primitive type of knee joint in currently living animals, the popliteus muscle attached directly to the fibular head. In marsupial species, the femorofibular meniscus was a pad of fibrocartilage that articulated with and was attached to the lateral femoral condyle and fibula. This meniscal structure had an attachment to the popliteus muscle and coursed in a groove on the lateral aspect of the lateral femoral condyle when the knee was in maximal flexion. He theorized that this femorofibular meniscus evolved over time to form the popliteus tendon and its attachment on the femur.

Last[14] reported that the popliteus complex emerged from underneath the "arcuate ligament" and that a very substantial portion of the popliteus muscle arose not from the tendon of the popliteus but from a portion of the arcuate ligament. A careful review of his illustrations demonstrates that the arcuate ligament that he was referring to was the popliteal aponeurosis to the lateral meniscus (**Fig. 2–2**). Last suggested that this attachment of the popliteus to the posterior aspect of the lateral meniscus helped to protect the lateral meniscus from injury. He also noted that fibrous strands directly connected the popliteus tendon to the lateral meniscus by synovial reflections above and below the meniscus. These are now known as the popliteomeniscal fascicles. In addition, he noted the popliteus tendon made a narrow groove in the posterolateral aspect of the lateral tibial plateau, just proximal to the fibular styloid. This bony landmark marks the location of the popliteus musculotendinous junction and is currently utilized to note the location of the popliteus tunnel for an anatomic posterolateral reconstruction (see Chapter 7).

Kaplan[20] reported that the popliteus tendon originated in front of and below the origin of the lateral collateral ligament (fibular collateral ligament) on the femur, and it was separated from the fibular collateral ligament by the joint capsule. He also stated that the popliteus tendon itself rarely adhered to the meniscus, and there was an intimate connection of the popliteus tendon to the fibular head by a ligament that connected both structures.[20,23,24] Kaplan reported that this connection sometimes reached the tibiofibular joint and was found in other species, including the chimpanzee. In this regard, he was referring to the popliteofibular ligament. Kaplan also noted that the muscular body of the popliteus, in contrast to

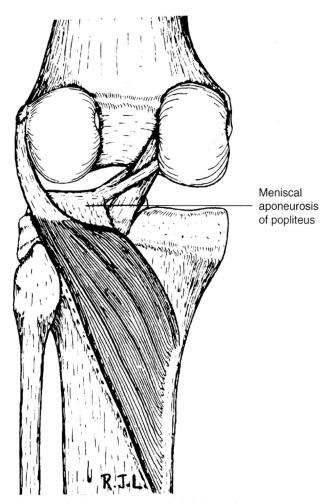

Figure 2–2   Posterior view of a left knee demonstrating the popliteus attachment to the posterior horn of the lateral meniscus (popliteal aponeurosis attachment to the lateral meniscus). (From Last RJ. The popliteus muscle and the lateral meniscus: with a note on the attachment of the medial meniscus. J Bone Joint Surg 1950;32B:93–99, with permission.)

Meniscal
aponeurosis
of popliteus

the popliteus tendon, adhered firmly to the lateral meniscus, the coronary ligament to the lateral meniscus, and the posterior capsule of the knee joint.[20,23,24] He reported that this attachment occurred through the means of a thick fascia, which he termed the popliteal fascia. We now know this to be the popliteal aponeurosis to the lateral meniscus. The relative immobility of the popliteus tendon at the knee was also noted by Kaplan, which he felt made this tendon a static stabilizer of the knee in all positions. He also noted the rare occurrence of a sesamoid bone, the cyamella, in the tendon of the popliteus in humans.[20] He also felt that the popliteus tendon was almost never adherent to the lateral meniscus (which we now know to be incorrect because of its popliteomeniscal fascicle attachments).[22,25] Kaplan[4] also noted that the meniscal remnant between the femur and the fibula in lower animal species eventually evolved into the popliteus tendon. In fact, he noted that the femoromeniscal ligament to the femorofibular meniscus appeared to have evolved into the popliteus attachment to the femur, whereas the meniscofibular ligament evolved into the popliteofibular ligament.

Lovejoy and Harden[26] reported that the popliteus had three attachments at the knee. They described them as attachments to the lateral femoral condyle, the fibular styloid (which we now know as the popliteofibular ligament), and the posterior horn of the lateral meniscus (the popliteal aponeurosis to the lateral meniscus). The femoral attachment was in a fossa that was anteroinferior to the lateral (fibular) collateral ligament. This fossa was the popliteus sulcus. They found a fibular attachment from the popliteus muscle to be present in all specimens (popliteofibular ligament). They noted that the femoral attachment, or the popliteus tendon, and the fibular attachment (popliteofibular ligament) formed the arms of a Y-shaped ligament that they stated had been previously described as a separate entity (**Fig. 2–3**). They reported that this separate entity

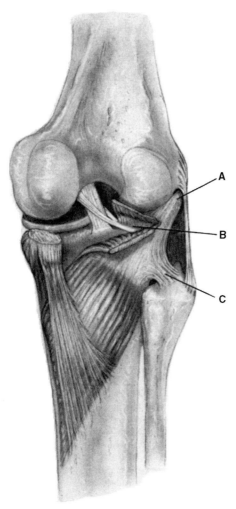

Figure 2–3   Illustration of the posterior view of a right knee demonstrating the Y-shaped ligament described by Lovejoy. A, popliteus femoral origin; B, popliteus aponeurosis to lateral meniscus; C, popliteofibular ligament. (From Lovejoy JF, Harden TT. Popliteus muscle in man. Anat Rec 1971;169:727–730, with permission.)

was incorrectly called the "arcuate" ligament. They felt that this was incorrect because this structure was not a distinct separate entity, but rather a distinct portion of the popliteus complex. However, their article was in the anatomy literature and thus not read by most orthopaedists, and so it was not well recognized at that time.

In 1975, Reis and de Carvalho[27] described the attachments of the human popliteus muscle complex at the knee. The proximal attachment of the popliteus muscle was in a depression just below the lateral epicondyle and was beneath and anterior and medial to the fibular collateral ligament's femoral attachment. They noted that the popliteus tendon had an oblique direction upward and downward, and formed approximately a 45-degree angle over the horizontal plane when it passed by the lateral tibial plateau. They concluded that the popliteus muscle had four attachments near the knee. They were the direct origin on the femur, the meniscal attachments, the attachments to the posterior capsule (popliteal aponeurosis), and the fibular head attachment (the popliteofibular ligament). They reported that the meniscal attachments (popliteomeniscal fascicles) united the popliteus tendon to the lateral meniscus and that the fibular attachment (the popliteofibular ligament) originated from the musculotendinous junction of the popliteus.

In 1979, Cohn and Mains[28] described the anatomy of the popliteal hiatus. They reported that the anatomy of the popliteus complex is constant at the popliteal hiatus. They observed two distinct ligamentous fascicles to the lateral meniscus: one for the superior surface and one for the inferior surface of the meniscus. These fascicles were noted to make up the floor and the roof of the popliteal hiatus, respectively. In carefully reviewing the authors' illustrations, one can see that the superior fascicle corresponds to what we now know as the posterosuperior popliteomeniscal fascicle, and the inferior fascicle corresponds to the anteroinferior popliteomeniscal fascicle.

Fabbriciani et al[5] reported in the Italian literature on the anatomy of the popliteus muscle complex of the knee in 1982. These authors reported that the popliteus muscle continued into a complex aponeurosis consisting of popliteocapsular (the popliteal aponeurosis to the lateral meniscus), popliteofibular, and popliteomeniscal (the popliteomeniscal fascicles) fibers. They reported that the popliteus developed into a strong tendon that attached on the lateral femoral condyle. They stated that there were both superior and inferior popliteomeniscal fibers (popliteomeniscal fascicles). In addition, they summarized some of the developmental phylogeny literature. They reported that comparative anatomy studies demonstrated that in lower order vertebrates, the fibula and the tibia each had a separate articulation with the femur with its respective meniscus. They also reported that the fibers of the popliteus muscle attached directly to the fibular head in lower animal species. As the fibular head descended distally in higher animal species, the differentiation of the meniscus between the femur and fibula was noted to occur. In the later stages of phylogenic development, they postulated the popliteus muscle became attached to the femorofibular meniscus, which evolved to become the popliteus tendon, and the popliteus muscle developed a tendinous attachment to the fibular head, which evolved to become the popliteofibular ligament. In addition, the popliteus tendon maintained its ties to the lateral meniscus (which we now refer to as the popliteal aponeurosis to the lateral meniscus and popliteomeniscal fascicles).

Seebacher et al[15] reported that the inner (deep) lamina of layer III (of the three anatomic layers that they described in their article) terminated posteriorly as a "Y-shaped arcuate" ligament, which spanned the junction between the popliteus muscle and its tendon from the fibular head to the femur. They stated that the superficial and inner lamina of layer III were always separated from each other in the region of the fibula by the inferior lateral genicular vessels (**Fig. 2–4**). They noted that the "arcuate" ligament inserted at the apex of the fibular styloid and was firmly adherent to the musculotendinous junction of the popliteus. They reported that in all cases a reinforcing structure was noted to course directly from the fibula to the popliteus musculotendinous junction. Seebacher et al also noted that a deep, or inner, lamina formed the hiatus for

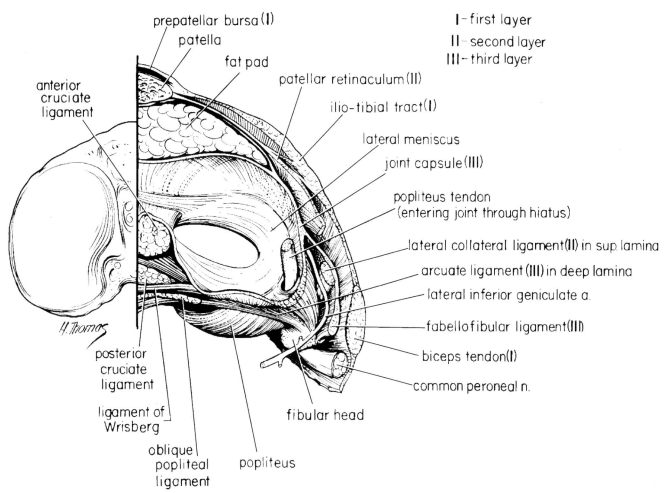

Figure 2–4 Axial illustration of a right knee with emphasis on the posterolateral knee structures. In this depiction, the authors note that the fabellofibular ligament and arcuate ligament (popliteofibular ligament) are separated from each other by the inferior lateral genicular artery. (From Seebacher JR, Inglis AE, Marshall JL, Warren RF. The structure of the posterolateral aspect of the knee. J Bone Joint Surg 1982;64A:536–541, with permission.)

the popliteus tendon (i.e., the popliteomeniscal fascicles). In understanding this work by Seebacher et al, it is important to note that a further anatomic study[29] from their center noted, in retrospect, that a direct attachment of the popliteus complex to the fibular head had not been recognized by Seebacher et al. These later researchers reported that they now understood this description to be the popliteofibular ligament. It is very important to recognize the group's retraction of the use of the term *arcuate ligament,* because the work of Seebacher et al[15] is still widely quoted in the orthopaedic and radiology literature.

The human embryonic development of the popliteus complex was described by Oransky and colleagues[30] in 1989. These authors found that the attachments of the popliteus complex to the lateral meniscus and its fibular head were formed during the process of embryonic cavitation during the formation of the popliteal hiatus. They found that this occurred at about the 10th week of embryonic development and it resulted in a separation of the popliteus tendon from the lateral meniscus. The popliteofibular ligament was found to develop soon after this. Oransky and colleagues also verified the location of the popliteofibular ligament in adult human cadavers and reported that it was a strong and constantly found structure in all specimens. They noted that it coursed between the posteromedial aspect of the fibular head and the lateral aspect of the popliteus tendon.

Another group of authors[16] reported on the popliteofibular ligament and found it to be present in 98% of their knee dissections. They reported that it was a short, strong, tendinous band that coursed between the popliteus tendon and the fibular styloid. They also stated that they believed that this structure should be considered a true distinct ligament of the knee joint with importance in preventing posterolateral rotation of the knee.

In the early 1990s, Stäubli and coauthors[22,25] reported extensively on the anatomy of the popliteus complex and its attachments to the lateral meniscus at the popliteal hiatus (**Fig. 2–5**). They noted that the popliteus tendon attachment on the femur was at the anterior aspect of the popliteal sulcus and anterior and distal to the lateral epicondyle in all cases. The popliteus tendon also caused a sinusoidal indentation of the articular cartilage where it crossed the lateral femoral condyle in extension, and only lay within the confines of the popliteal sulcus when the knee was significantly flexed. The anteroinferior popliteomeniscal fascicle was always present and blended into the middle third of the lateral meniscus. This fascicle created the anterior floor of the popliteal hiatus that can be seen arthroscopically. The posterosuperior popliteomeniscal fascicle was also found to blend into the posterior horn of the lateral meniscus and the meniscofemoral portion of the posterior capsule of the joint. Stäubli and coauthors also described the popliteofibular fascicle (ligament), which consisted of anterior and posterior divisions. They reported that it arose from the proximal tibiofibular joint and fibular styloid region and extended to the musculotendinous junction of the popliteus. They reported the popliteofibular ligament had the shape of an inverted Y and consisted of an anterior division that blended proximally into the anteroinferior popliteomeniscal fascicle and a posterior division that attached to the posterior aspect of the fibular styloid and was adjacent and adherent to the proximal tibiofibular joint capsule. They also reported that the inferior lateral genicular artery passed posterior to the

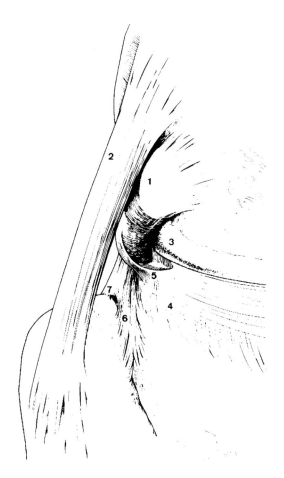

Figure 2–5   The popliteus complex and its relationship to the lateral meniscus and fibula in a right knee. 1, popliteus tendon; 2, fibular collateral ligament; 3, sulcus statarius; 4, meniscotibial portion of mid-third lateral capsule ligament; 5, anteroinferior popliteomeniscal fascicles; 6, anterior division of popliteofibular ligament; 7, posterior division of popliteofibular ligament. (From Stäubli HU, Birrer S. The popliteus tendon and its fascicles at the popliteus hiatus: gross anatomy and functional arthroscopic evaluation with and without anterior cruciate ligament deficiency. Arthroscopy 1990;6:209–220, with permission.)

popliteofibular ligament and anterior to the fabellofibular ligament and its associated structures.

Watanabe et al[31] reported that the popliteofibular ligament was present in 93% of their dissected knee specimens. They reported that the popliteus tendon attachment on the femur was consistently present at the popliteal sulcus. They also did three-dimensional geometry studies of the popliteus tendon with varying degrees of knee flexion by inserting metal markers into the anterior and posterior aspect of the popliteus tendon and obtaining radiographs. They found that the anterior part of the popliteus tendon became tighter with higher knee flexion angles and the posterior part of the popliteus tendon became tighter near extension. From this information, they theorized that the posterior aspect of the popliteus tendon and the popliteofibular ligament would act as restraints near full extension, whereas the anterior portion of the popliteus tendon would act as a posterolateral rotatory restraint with increasing knee flexion.

Maynard and coauthors[29] also reported on the anatomy of the popliteofibular ligament. Their dissection technique helped to isolate it better than most previous techniques in the past. They dissected their specimens from inside the joint to outside rather than the usual outside-in technique. By this method, they were able to isolate the popliteofibular ligament better than did previous dissection techniques. These authors found the popliteofibular ligament to be substantial in size and present in all of their dissected knees. The popliteofibular ligament fibers were noted to fuse to the popliteus tendon and to diverge to the proximal and posterior aspect of the fibular head. These authors were noted to be from the same research center as Seebacher et al[15] and Gollehon et al,[32] and they were able to report in retrospect that their center's previous work did not recognize that the direct attachment from the popliteus complex to the fibular head, that is, the popliteofibular ligament, existed when their earlier studies were performed.

Sussman and coauthors[33] also reported on a study on the human fetal development of the popliteomeniscal fascicles. They reported that at 23 weeks of gestation, fetal knees were noted to have the same morphologic characteristic structures as human adult knees. The lateral meniscus and the popliteus tendon were noted to be held together by the anteroinferior and posterosuperior popliteomeniscal fascicles.

In summarizing the literature on the popliteus complex at the knee, it can be clearly seen that the main confusion lies with the structures that course from the fibular head and styloid region to the popliteus muscle and tendon. The femoral attachment of the popliteus tendon on the popliteal sulcus at the femur[1,2,5,6,14,20–22,25–28,30,31] has been found to be consistently identified in the same anatomic location by multiple authors.

Although some authors have failed to note the presence[20] or the universal occurrence[14] of the popliteomeniscal fascicles, it appears that this oversight was primarily due to a lack of detailed dissection or anecdotal information rather than based on a large number of dissections detailing these structures. Stäubli and coauthors[22,25] reported on these three popliteomeniscal fascicles, which have been defined to be the anteroinferior, posterosuperior, and posteroinferior popliteomeniscal fascicles. Although others have also reported on these fascicles,[5,18,20,27,28,30,33] they have not reported on these structures in as much detail as Stäubli's group.

The primary reason for confusion about the anatomy of the posterolateral corner of the knee is the varied nomenclature of the popliteofibular ligament. Many authors over a long period of time have noted the presence of a popliteofibular ligament, also called the popliteal attachment to the fibular head.[1,2,5,16,20–27,29–31] However, this structure was omitted from the update of the *Nomina Anatomica* by the International Congress of Anatomists.[13] Thus, many authors did not formally recognize it, and it resulted in many different names given to the structure.[15] One of the most commonly quoted anatomic descriptions, by Seebacher et al,[15] reported that the innermost (deep) lamina of their posterolateral structures, which they named a "Y-shaped arcuate ligament," spanned the junction between the fibular head and popliteus and was anterior to the inferior lateral genicular artery. Seebacher et al's description of a Y-shaped arcuate ligament is almost identical to the description provided by Stäubli and Birrer[22] for the popliteofibular ligament. In addition, their description of this structure in relation to the inferior lateral genicular artery would confirm they were actually referring to the popliteofibular ligament. As I have mentioned previously, another previous publication from the same research center as Seebacher's, which reported on the anatomy of the popliteofibular ligament in detail,[29] noted that these and other previous studies[15,32] did not recognize the existence of the popliteofibular ligament at that point in time and named it the "arcuate ligament." Thus, in summary, it would appear that the existence of the popliteofibular ligament has been noted by many authors all along, and the confusion regarding this lack of recognition now appears to be resolved.

◆ Biceps Femoris Complex at the Knee

Vallois[34] performed extensive comparative anatomy studies of the primate knee. In all primates but humans, he noted that the biceps femoris complex ended distally as a fascial attachment to the fascia lata and anterior compartment musculature of the leg without any direct attachment to the fibula.

Last[18] reported that the lateral ligament, or fibular collateral ligament, separated the biceps tendon into superficial and deep parts. The deep part of the tendon coursed between the fibular collateral ligament and the lateral joint capsule and is now known as the anterior arm of the short head of the biceps femoris. The superficial portion of the biceps tendon was noted to wrap around the fibular collateral ligament, attach to the fibular head, and send an expansion over the anteromedial tibia.

Sneath[35] also reported on the attachments of the biceps femoris at the knee in a dissection of multiple knees. He reported that the long head of the biceps femoris attached to the fibular head, the lateral ligament of the knee, and the lateral tibial plateau. Proximal to the primary attachments of the common biceps tendon, he noted that the biceps tendon blended anteriorly with the iliotibial tract and gave off an expansion to the fascia covering the anterior, lateral, and posterior compartments of the leg. Sneath also reported that the remaining distal portion of the biceps tendon, primarily derived from the short head of the biceps, had three lamina (**Fig. 2–6**). The superficial lamina passed superficial, or lateral, to the fibular collateral ligament and attached to the lateral tibial plateau. This structure is now known as the anterior arm of the long head of the biceps femoris. The intermediate lamina blended with the posterior border of the distal third of the lateral ligament and is now known as the lateral aponeurotic attachments of the long and short heads of the biceps femoris to the fibular collateral ligament. The deep lamina passed deep, or medial, to the fibular collateral ligament and inserted onto the lateral tibial plateau of the tibia immediately posterior to the iliotibial band. This is currently known as the

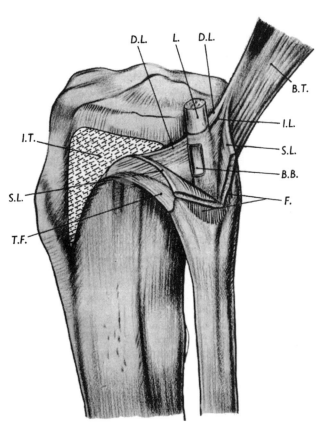

Figure 2–6   The lateral view of the left knee demonstrating the deep lamina biceps bursa (BB), biceps tendon (BT), (the anterior arm of the short head of the biceps femoris) (DL), Fibular collateral liqment (F), intermediate lamina (lateral aponeurosis of the long and short heads of the biceps femoris) (IL), fibular collateral ligament (L), superficial lamina (the anterior arm of the long head of the biceps femoris) (SL) and tibiofibular joint (TF). (From Sneath RS. The insertion of the biceps femoris. J Anat 1955;89:550–553, with permission.)

anterior arm of the short head of the biceps femoris. He also noted that there was a constant bursa (the fibular collateral ligament–biceps femoris bursa) that separated the fibular collateral ligament from the superficial and deep lamina of the biceps tendon. In other words, he was reporting that this bursa separated the anterior arms of the short and long heads of the biceps femoris from each other, which we now know to be somewhat true as the biceps bursa has the fibular head as a portion of its medial border.

Kaplan[20,36] reported that the biceps femoris tendon had an attachment to the iliotibial band, and the biceps femoris connected distally onto the anterior compartment of the leg. These layers are now known as the reflected arm of the long head of the biceps femoris for the iliotibial band attachment and the anterior aponeurosis of the long head of the biceps femoris for the fascial attachment over the anterior compartment of the leg. Kaplan also observed that the fibular attachment of the biceps femoris muscle surrounded the fibular attachment of the lateral collateral ligament with a bursa, which is now called the fibular collateral ligament–biceps femoris bursa.[37] Kaplan also noted that there was an intimate attachment between the fascia of the iliotibial band and biceps femoris near the fibular head,[20] which is now called the confluence with the capsulo-osseous layer of the iliotibial band.[38,39] Kaplan[36] also noted that there was an anterior extension of the biceps femoris to the proximolateral tibia, which was medial to the fibular collateral ligament, which is now known as the anterior arm of the short head of the biceps femoris.

In a series of dissections on 10 fresh and 21 embalmed knees, Marshall et al[8] found that the fleshy fibers of the long head of the biceps femoris formed a broad flat tendon about 7 to 10 cm proximal to the knee joint. The short head of the biceps femoris was found to join the tendon of the long head at its undersurface, remaining fleshy almost to the fibular head, at which point the two structures joined to form a thick short tendon. Marshall et al reported that just before it reached the lateral collateral ligament, the common biceps femoris tendon split into three different layers: superficial, middle, and deep. The superficial layer was lateral to the lateral collateral ligament, the middle layer surrounded it, and the deep layer was medial and deep to the lateral collateral ligament. In this regard, their three layers were similar to the three layers of the biceps femoris described by Sneath.[35] Marshall et al reported that the superficial layer formed three expansions. Their description of different layers and expansions within layers makes it very difficult to follow their work. The first of these expansions was a thin and sheet-like anterior expansion that extended distal to the lateral collateral ligament and blended with the superficial fascia over the anterior compartment of the leg. We now know this as the anterior aponeurosis of the long head of the biceps femoris. They also reported that some of the deep fibers of the superificial layer inserted onto the lateral aspect of the fibular head, and this is now known as the anterior arm of the long head of the biceps femoris. The middle expansion of the superficial layer that Marshall et al described had attachments to the fibular head (the anterior arm of the long head of the biceps femoris) and blended distally with the fascia over the peroneal muscles (now called the anterior aponeurosis of the long head of the biceps femoris). The posterior expansion of this superficial layer extended posterodistally and blended with the fascia over the calf muscles. This is now known as the distal fascial expansion of the long head of the biceps femoris.

Marshall et al[8] also observed that the middle layer of the common biceps tendon was a thin, poorly defined layer that surrounded and attached posterior to the distal fourth of the lateral collateral ligament like a sling. They reported that this layer split to surround the lateral collateral ligament and was separated from the ligament by a bursa. We now know these layers to be the anterior arm of the long head of the biceps femoris and lateral aponeurotic attachments of the long and short head of the biceps femoris to the fibular collateral ligament. The bursa that Marshall et al described is also known as the fibular collateral ligament–biceps femoris bursa.[37]

Marshall et al[8] also stated that the deep layer of the distal aspect of the common biceps tendon bifurcated and had fibular and tibial attachments (**Fig. 2–7**). The tibial attachment was just posterior to Gerdy's tubercle and is now called the anterior arm of the short head of the biceps femoris. The fibular attachment was to the fibular styloid process and the upper surface of the fibular head and is referred to currently as the direct arms of the long and short head of the biceps femoris. Marshall et al also described a well-developed

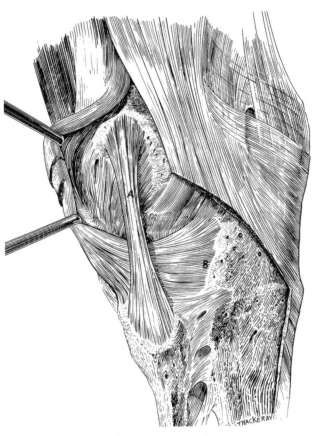

Figure 2–7   Lateral illustration of a right knee with the superficial layer of the iliotibial band and lateral aspects of the long biceps removed. The deep layer of the biceps femoris (the anterior arm of the short head of the biceps femoris) (B) is noted to pass medial to the fibular collateral ligament (A). In addition, it was noted to have an attachment on the posterolateral aspect of the fibular styloid (direct arm of the short head of the biceps femoris). The capsular expansion (capsular arm of the short head of the biceps femoris) is noted to be present just medial to the distal retractor in the illustration. (From Marshall JL, Girgis FG, Zelko RR. The biceps femoris tendon and its functional significance. J Bone Joint Surg 1972;54A:1444–1450, with permission.)

fascial expansion from the biceps femoris to the posterolateral aspect of the knee joint capsule, which is now called the capsular arm of the short head of the biceps femoris.

Seebacher et al[15] reported that the superficial portion of layer I of the three layers of their dissections included the superficial portion of the biceps femoris and its posterior expansion. They also reported that just posterior to the iliotibial tract, the superficial lamina of layer III of their description, which is now believed to have included the lateral aponeurosis of the long and short heads of the biceps femoris and the capsular arm of the short head of the biceps femoris, surrounded the lateral collateral ligament and ended posteriorly at the fabellofibular ligament, or its analogue, the short lateral ligament, in the absence of a fabella.

Terry and LaPrade[38] performed anatomic dissections on 30 fresh-frozen cadaveric knees and described the main components of the long and short heads of the biceps femoris of the knee. Their nomenclature for the biceps femoris is the nomenclature adapted in Chapter 3 on the anatomy of the posterolateral knee.

In addition, LaPrade and Hamilton[37] reported on the quantitative anatomy of the fibular collateral ligament–biceps femoris bursa. Although this bursa had been noted to be present by several other authors,[8,20,35,38] its location, size, shape, and prevalence had not been reported on previously. The fibular collateral ligament–biceps bursa was noted to be located over the distal 25% of the fibular collateral ligament and formed an inverted J shape over the anterior and anterolateral portions of the fibular collateral ligament and was noted to be present in all knees. Its lateral border was the anterior arm of the long head of the biceps femoris.

In summarizing the previous literature on the anatomy of the long and short heads of the biceps femoris, the majority of the various components of the biceps femoris complex have been described before, but no single article described all the individual components of both the long and short heads of the biceps femoris until the work by Terry and LaPrade.[38] The components of the long head of the biceps that were described previously included the reflected arm,[20,35,36] direct arm,[7,8,18,35] lateral aponeurotic expansion,[15,18,35] anterior arm,[7,8,18,35] distal fascial expansion,[8,35] and anterior aponeurotic expansion.[18,20,35] In a similar fashion, previous descriptions of the components of the short head of the biceps femoris included the proximal muscular attachment of the short head to the long head,[35] biceps–capsulo-osseous iliotibial band confluence,[8,20,40,41] capsular arm,[8,15] direct arm,[7,8,18,35] lateral aponeurotic expansion,[15,18,35] and the anterior arm.[8,18,35,36] In spite of the fact that different authors described these different components of the biceps femoris of the knee, there was no significant difference in the descriptions of these varying structures among the various authors and reporting institutions. I also believe that it is clear that describing these complex structures by a layered approach, rather than by descriptive anatomy based on their course and attachments, is much more difficult to understand and remember.

◆ Iliotibial Band at the Knee

Maissiat[9] was one of the first to report on the anatomy and function of the iliotibial band in a monogram in 1843. He reported that the "ilio-trochantero-tibiale bande" (iliotibial band) was only present in humans. In the 19th century, the iliotibial band was commonly referred to as the "band of Maissiat." Gerdy[42] also was one of the first to describe the iliotibial band at the knee. He reported that it inserted on a prominence on the lateral aspect of the proximal tibia. Segond[43] later named this attachment site as "the tubercle of Gerdy." It is through Segond's work that we still refer to the attachment site of the iliotibial band on the tibia as Gerdy's tubercle. Segond also reported on a pearly fibrous band of the iliotibial band that coursed from the posterolateral aspect of the knee and attached just behind Gerdy's tubercle. This is what is now called the capsulo-osseous layer of the iliotibial band of the knee.[40]

Last[18] reported that the iliotibial band was a ribbon-like condensation of the fascial lata. He reported that it attached distally to a prominent facet on the lateral tibial plateau, which is now called Gerdy's tubercle.

Kaplan[20] stated that when a surgeon made a straight oblique incision over the lateral side of the knee, the first fascial layer encountered was the fascia lata, which we now call the superficial layer of the iliotibial band. Kaplan also stated that this "fascia lata" adhered intimately to the lateral supracondylar tubercle and blended into the lateral intermuscular septum. These layers are now called the deep and capsulo-osseous layers of the iliotibial band and are also commonly called "Kaplan's fibers." Kaplan also reported that fascia from the iliotibial band adhered to the biceps femoris over the fibular head, which is now called the confluence with the capsulo-osseous layer of the iliotibial band. The iliotibial band was described as a thickening of the fascia lata, running from the base of the greater trochanter to the lateral tibial tubercle (Gerdy's tubercle). Kaplan also reported that the anterior portion of the iliotibial band curved anteriorly and blended with the lateral aspect of the patella. This is now called the iliopatellar band portion of the iliotibial band.

In a separate article, Kaplan[7] reported in more detail on the anatomy of the iliotibial band. He reported that the structure was also known as the iliotibial tract or band of Maissiat. As part of the study, Kaplan performed comparative anatomy dissections to study the anatomy of the iliotibial band in other animal species and the human knee. He found that even in higher-level primates, such as the gibbon, orangutan, and gorilla, there was no iliotibial band present. He noted that only in the human lower extremity was there an open space between the biceps femoris tendon and the vastus lateralis muscle at the knee joint, which permitted passage of the iliotibial band to insert onto Gerdy's tubercle. Kaplan also noted that the distal aspect of the iliotibial band was intimately connected to the lateral intermuscular septum and the linea aspera in the region of the supracondylar tubercle of the lateral femoral condyle. We now call these structures Kaplan's fibers and they consist of the deep and capsulo-osseous layers of the iliotibial band. Kaplan also reported that the anterior portion of the iliotibial band was connected by curved fibers to the lateral aspect of the patella, which we now know as the iliopatellar band.

Seebacher et al[15] reported that layer I of the three layers of their dissection descriptions of the posterolateral knee structures was a superficial layer and consisted of two parts. One of these two parts included the iliotibial band, now called the superficial layer of the iliotibial band.

Terry et al[40] reported on the anatomy of the iliopatellar and iliotibial bands of the knee. Their description of the anatomy of the iliotibial band follows the nomenclature currently adapted to describe these structures. The superficial layer of the iliotibial band was defined as the superficial fascial layer that covered the lateral aspect of the knee. The iliopatellar band consisted of the fibers that curved anteriorly from the main vertically oriented fibers of the iliotibial band and attached to the lateral border of the patella. Two additional layers were also described, which were deep, or medial, to the superificial layer of the

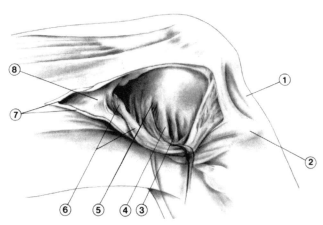

Figure 2–8 Lateral illustration of a right knee demonstrating the relationships of the deep layer[8] and capsulo-osseous layer[8] of the iliotibial band. 1, patellar tendon; 2, Gerdy's tubercle; 3, fibular collateral ligament; 4, lateral gastrocnemius tendon; 5, plantaris muscle; 6, capsulo-osseous layer of iliotibial band; 7, cut edges of superficial layer of iliotibial band; 8, deep layer of iliotibial band. (From Terry GC, Hughston JC, Norwood LA. The anatomy of the iliopatellar band and iliotibial tract. Am J Sports Med 1986;14:39–45, with permission.)

iliotibial band (**Fig. 2–8**). One of these was the deep layer. The deep layer of the iliotibial band extended in a curvilinear fashion in the coronal plane, following the lateral outline of the lateral femoral condyle, from the distal termination of the lateral intermuscular septum, and attached slightly distal on the medial border of the superficial layer. The capsulo-osseous layer of the iliotibial band was also described as the medial wall of the deep layer of the iliotibial band, which functioned as an anterolateral ligament of the knee as it formed a sling over the lateral femoral condyle. The capsulo-osseous layer of the iliotibial band was medial and distal to the deep layer. This capsulo-osseous layer also had a proximal origin continuous with the fascia over the posterolateral aspects of the lateral gastrocnemius and plantaris muscles and also to the supracondylar area of the femur. It then coursed distal and lateral to where it attached to the tibia just posterior to Gerdy's tubercle. They also noted that the capsulo-osseous layer had an attachment to the fascia from the short head of the biceps femoris along its course, called the confluence of the short head of the biceps femoris with the capsulo-osseous layer, which formed a sling, in the coronal plane, along the lateral aspect of the knee. This capsulo-osseous layer was the sling that was reconstructed in extraarticular anterior cruciate ligament reconstructions.

In 1987, Lobenhoffer et al[41] reported on the anatomy of the attachments of the iliotibial band at the distal femur. They described a supracondylar bundle that coursed proximomedially from the superficial layer of the iliotibial band and attached to the supracondylar area of the femur. This supracondylar bundle is also known as the deep layer of the iliotibial band. In addition, Lobenhoffer et al noted that there were concurrent fibers that coursed between the superficial layer of the iliotibial band and the lateral intramuscular septum at the distal dorsolateral femur. They also reported that a fibrous tract of the iliotibial band curved over the lateral aspect of the knee joint and connected with Gerdy's tubercle to form a concurrent attachment between the tibial and dorsolateral femur. We know this now to be the capsulo-osseous layer of the iliotibial band. The femoral attachments of these tracts were along the femur just distal to the termination of the lateral intramuscular septum and the medial attachment of the supracondylar bundle (deep layer of the iliotibial band). They reported that these fibers had a lateral arched fiber arrangement with a reversed course in relation to the other insertions of the iliotibial band at the femur. It appears what they meant in their description of a "reverse course" was that it attached distally along the superficial layer of the iliotibial band and coursed much more proximally compared with the supracondylar bundle, or deep layer of the iliotibial band, to attach the femur. Thus, Lobenhoffer et al called these structures the "retrograde fiber tracks," which correspond to the capsulo-osseous layer of the iliotibial band (**Fig. 2–9**). They also reported that there were connections from these retrograde track fibers (capsulo-osseous layer) to the biceps tendon (confluence of the capsulo-osseous layer of the iliotibial band of the short head of the biceps femoris).

In summarizing the literature on the anatomy of the iliotibial band, it should be noted that the terms *iliotibial band* and *iliotibial tract* have been used interchangeably in the past.[7] The most commonly used term over time has been the *iliotibial band.* The superficial layer of the iliotibial band, which is the main fascial layer, and its distal attachment to Gerdy's tubercle, has been noted to be present by multiple authors.[7,9,15,18,20,40–43] Although he did not describe the attachment of the superficial layer of the iliotibial band to the distolateral femur in great detail, Kaplan[7,20] appears to be the first to describe these deep attachments. This is the reason that these attachments are commonly called "Kaplan's fibers."[41,44] In addition, the iliopatellar band has also been described by both Kaplan[20] and Terry et al.[40]

Both Terry et al[40] and Lobenhoffer et al[41] independently described the two deep structures that connect the medial attachment of the superficial layer of

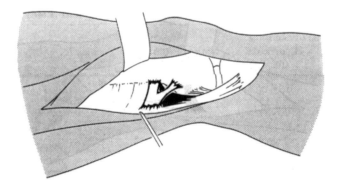

Figure 2–9 Lateral illustration of a right knee, with the superficial layer of the iliotibial band retracted, to demonstrate the course and attachment of the "retrograde fiber tracks" (capsulo-osseous layer of the iliotibial band) from an attachment just distal to the lateral intermuscular septum on the femur (outlined in dark black) to course distally to attach just posterior to Gerdy's tubercle. (From Lobenhoffer P, Posel P, Witt S, Piehler J, Wirth CJ. Distal femoral fixation of the iliotibial tract. Arch Orthop Trauma Surg 1987;106:285–290, with permission.)

the iliotibial band to the distolateral aspect of the femur. Although it appears that both groups of authors disagree slightly on the femoral attachment sites of these structures, they do agree that the deep layer,[40] or the supracondylar bundle,[41] attaches to the femur in a more transverse manner, whereas the "deeper" and more distal capsulo-osseous,[40] or retrograde fiber tract,[41] layer forms an anterolateral sling of tissue over the anterolateral aspect of the knee around the lateral aspect of the lateral femoral condyle to attach just posterior to Gerdy's tubercle on the tibia. It has been noted that this lateral sling of tissue from the iliotibial band is what most surgeons attempted to reconstruct in extraarticular anterior cruciate ligament reconstructions.

◆ Mid-Third Lateral Capsular Ligament

Hughston et al[45] reported that the mid-third lateral capsular ligament was a strong and major static support against lateral forces at 30 degrees of knee flexion over the lateral aspect of the knee. It was noted to attach proximally to the lateral epicondyle and distally to attach along the midlateral joint margin of the tibia.

Johnson[44] reported that the lateral capsular ligament complex attached in the horizontal plane to the lateral meniscus. He also noted that this complex had vertical attachments to bone, ligaments, and tendons. He noted that the central portion of the lateral capsule, or mid-third lateral capsular ligament, had thicker fibers, and its attachment to the lateral tibial plateau was strong.

Seebacher et al[15] also noted that the lateral capsular ligament, or the midlateral capsule (or mid-third lateral capsular ligament), was very strong at the point of fusion of the superficial and deep lamina of the layer III of their three layers of their posterolateral knee dissections. Seebacher et al also felt that its strength was responsible for the avulsion of tibial metaphyseal bone seen in lateral knee injuries (Segond fractures).[43]

Terry and LaPrade[38] noted that the anterior arm of the short head of the biceps femoris had a common attachment with this meniscotibial portion of the mid-third lateral capsular ligament. In most instances, both structures were commonly found attached to a Segond avulsion fracture or soft tissue avulsion off of the proximolateral tibia.

To summarize, it has been recognized that the mid-third lateral capsular ligament is a thickening of the central portion of the lateral portion. Its tibial, or meniscotibial, portion has been noted to be attached to Segond fractures.[15,20,44]

◆ Oblique Popliteal Ligament

The oblique popliteal ligament, which appears to have been first described by Winslow,[46] has been noted to be an expansion off the semimembranosus muscle over the posterior aspect of the knee. The oblique popliteal ligament develops later in fetal life and has been noted to be present as a thick fibrous band at between 30 and 32 weeks of fetal development.[19] Several literature sources have noted the lateral attachment site of the oblique popliteal ligament to be to the posterior aspect of the lateral femoral condyle,[18,20,46,47] whereas others have indicated an attachment to the lateral capsule.[4,15,45,48–53] Seebacher et al[15] and Müller[53] noted that the lateral attachment of the oblique popliteal ligament was to a cartilaginous or a bony fabella. Kaplan[4] noted that the oblique popliteal ligament was a wide band that coursed from the tibial attachment of the semimembranosus tendon toward the origin of the lateral gastrocnemius complex over the lateral femoral condyle. Kaplan also reported that the oblique popliteal ligament was always present, and its lateral border arched over the popliteus muscle and formed the medial arch of the arcuate ligament. In comparative anatomy studies, the oblique popliteal ligament was also noted to be present in the mountain gorilla.[54]

◆ Coronary Ligament of the Lateral Meniscus

Last[14] described the coronary ligament and noted that it attached the inferior border of the lateral meniscus to the edge of the articular cartilage of the tibia. He reported that it was deep to the overlying popliteal attachment to the lateral meniscus, also called the popliteal aponeurosis to the lateral meniscus, and was part of a true capsule of the knee joint (**Fig. 2–10**). Kaplan[20] reported that the coronary ligament of the lateral meniscus was deep to the inferior lateral genicular artery over the

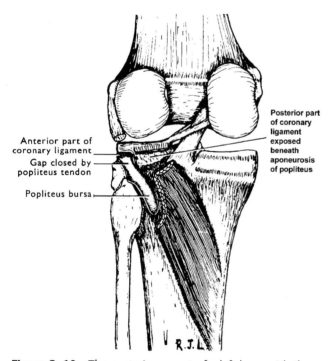

Anterior part of coronary ligament

Gap closed by popliteus tendon

Popliteus bursa

Posterior part of coronary ligament exposed beneath aponeurosis of popliteus

Figure 2–10   The posterior aspect of a left knee with the popliteal aponeurosis to the lateral meniscus removed to expose the coronary ligament to the lateral meniscus. (From Last RJ. The popliteus muscle and the lateral meniscus: with a note on the attachment of the medial meniscus. J Bone Joint Surg 1950;32B:93–99, with permission.)

posterior and lateral aspect of the knee. Seebacher et al[15] also reported that the coronary ligament was the capsular attachment to the outer edge of the lateral meniscus and was formed by layer III of the three layers of their posterolateral knee dissection. In addition, Stäubli and Birrer[22] noted that the coronary ligament was the meniscotibial portion of the posterior capsule to the lateral meniscus.

In summary, the literature supports the nomenclature of the coronary ligament as the meniscotibial portion of the posterior capsule, which attaches the posterior aspect of the lateral meniscus to the posterior aspect of the tibia.[14,15,20,22]

◆ Lateral Gastrocnemius Tendon

Haines[6] reported on comparative anatomy studies of the lateral gastrocnemius muscle and tendon complex. He noted that they were present in marsupials, and part of this tendon was noted to originate off the sesamoid bone, called the fabella, which served as a common partial attachment for the lateral gastrocnemius and plantaris muscles.

Kaplan[20] observed that the lateral head of the gastrocnemius muscle originated from the lateral femoral condyle just above the origin of the lateral collateral ligament and also from the thick capsule of the joint. This capsule was very thick under the lateral gastrocnemius complex. Stäubli noted in his cryosectioned dissections of the posterolateral aspect of the knee that the lateral gastrocnemius tendon blended into the proximal portion of the posterior meniscofemoral capsule. In addition, Stäubli[55] reported that the lateral gastrocnemius muscle acted to tension the posterior capsule and to passively control hyperextension of the knee due to the intimate attachment where it blended into the posterior aspect of the capsule.

◆ Fabellofibular Ligament

Weitbrecht,[56] a German anatomist, reported on the presence of the short lateral ligament, which attached to the lowest part of the lateral femoral condyle, or its little bone (the fabella), and then coursed to the tip of the fibula. He also reported that the short lateral ligament ended proximally along the posterolateral capsule of the joint and not directly on the femur. His illustration, which was reproduced in Kaplan's[4] work, demonstrates that he was referring to the fabellofibular ligament (**Fig. 2–11**).

The French anatomist Dujarier[57] described the peroneosesamoid ligament of the knee joint in 1905. In this review, he was referring to the fabellofibular ligament. Dujarier reported that the anterior portion of the fibular portion of the arcuate ligament, which coursed from the fibula to the sesamoid bone of the lateral gastrocnemius (the fabella), formed a fairly resistant ligament that he called the short external lateral ligament. Based on his descriptions, we now see that he was referring to the fabellofibular ligament.

Last[18] reported that the short lateral ligament constituted both the "arcuate" ligament (popliteofibular ligament and popliteal aponeurosis to the lateral

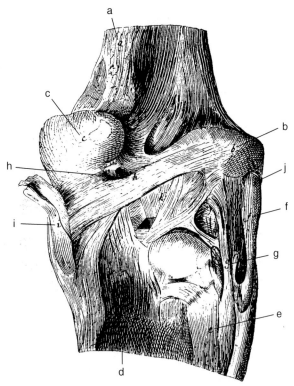

Figure 2–11   Illustration reproduced from Weitbrecht (1742) of the posterior aspect of the right knee. a, femur; b, lateral femoral condyle; c, medial femoral condyle; d, tibia; e, fibular; f, long external lateral ligament (fibular collateral ligament), g, short lateral ligament (fabellofibular ligament). h, oblique popliteal ligament; i, semimembanosus tendon; j, membranous expansion: (From Kaplan EB. The fabellofibular and short lateral ligaments of the knee joint. J Bone Joint Surg 1961;43A:169–179, with permission.)

meniscus) and the structure that coursed from the fibular styloid to the lateral epicondyle. It would appear from his illustrations that the short external lateral ligament in his description constituted the popliteofibular ligament and the lateral aspect of the popliteus tendon and not the fabellofibular ligament. Last[14] also reported that the "powerful" short external lateral ligament functioned to reinforce the lateral ligament (fibular collateral ligament) (**Fig. 2–12**).

Kaplan[4] reported that the fabellofibular ligament was "the short lateral ligament" of the knee joint, which had been described in articles in the previous literature.[56,57] He reported it had also been described as a short lateral ligament by Vallois.[34] Kaplan reported that he had reviewed the literature and found that the short lateral ligament was described mostly as a part of the lateral arch of the "arcuate" ligament, or as a reinforcement of the posterior capsule. This reinforcement of the posterior capsule is now known as the capsular arm of the short head of the biceps femoris. Although there have been multiple names given to this ligament in the past, such as the short external lateral ligament, the short lateral ligament, and the peroneosesamoid ligament, Kaplan named this structure the fabellofibular ligament due its course between the fibula and fabella.

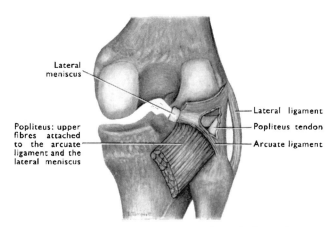

Lateral meniscus

Popliteus: upper fibres attached to the arcuate ligament and the lateral meniscus

Lateral ligament

Popliteus tendon

Arcuate ligament

Figure 2–12 The posterior aspect of a right knee demonstrating the course of Last's description of an arcuate ligament (popliteofibular ligament) from its attachment on the fibular head and styloid to its attachment to the popliteal musculotendinous junction and to its adherence to the posterior aspect of the lateral meniscus (popliteal aponeurosis to the lateral meniscus). (From Last RJ. Some anatomical details of the knee joint. J Bone Joint Surg 1948;30B:683–688, with permission.)

Kaplan[4] stated that the fabellofibular ligament was strongest in the kangaroo and in those animal species where the function and size of the gastrocnemius muscle was most important. He observed that in the absence of a bony fabella, a short lateral ligament represented a homologue of the fabellofibular ligament. Kaplan also observed that when a bony fabella was present, the size of the fabellofibular ligament was much larger than a short lateral ligament with no bony fabella. He also reported that the fabellofibular ligament attached on the fabella between the plantaris and the lateral gastrocnemius muscles and coursed to the tip of the fibular styloid, just posterior to the biceps tendon attachment. This is now known as the direct arm attachment of the short head of the biceps femoris. Kaplan reported that the fabellofibular ligament was posterior to the inferior lateral genicular artery. He theorized that the fabellofibular ligament may be a structure in involution in humans. He felt that both of these structures, the fabellofibular ligament and the short lateral ligament, depending on the presence of a fabella, represented a fourth ligamentous structure that contributed to lateral knee stability when it was in extension. The other structures were the iliotibial band, the fibular collateral ligament, and the popliteus tendon.

Seebacher et al[15] noted that the superficial lamina of layer III of the three layers of their posterolateral knee dissections ended posteriorly at a variably sized fabellofibular ligament or its homologue, the short external ligament. They reported on differing variations in the size of the fabellofibular ligament depending on whether there was a bony fabella, where the fabellofibular ligament was usually noted to be robust; a cartilaginous fabella, where the fabellofibular ligament was of modest size; or no palpable fabella (in 13% of knees), where a reinforcing fibrous structure was present over the capsule in this region. We now recognize that this structure corresponds with the capsular arm of the short head of the biceps femoris. In all cases, the fabellofibular or short external ligament was reported to attach to the apex of the fibular styloid and ascended vertically to attach to the lateral gastrocnemius at the fabella, where it was joined by the lateral attachment of the oblique popliteal ligament.

Müller[53] noted that the fabellofibular ligament was a portion of the "arcuate" ligament complex that coursed from the fibula to the fabella. The fabella was noted to be located at a point where multiple stresses on the knee intersected. The structures located at this point included the oblique popliteal ligament, lateral gastrocnemius tendon, and the fabellofibular ligament.

Sudasna and Harnsiriwattanagit[16] performed anatomic dissections on 50 formalin-preserved cadavers and reported that the fabellofibular ligament, or its homologue the short lateral ligament (in the absence of a bony fabella), was present in 72% of their dissected knees. They noted that in the 68% of knees with a palpable fabella, the ligament was long and slender. In the other 4% of knees, the ligament was wider and attached to the lateral femoral condyle, close to the origin of the lateral head of the gastrocnemius. They noted that the size of the fabellofibular ligament was small, and they postulated that it could not play a major role as a static stabilizer of the knee. They also reported that they did not find it to be as large in their dissections as it had been described by Last[14] or Kaplan.[4] We now know that Last was actually referring to the popliteofibular ligament and not the fabellofibular ligament, whereas Kaplan was referring to the fabellofibular ligament. It should also be noted that thin fibrous structures, such as the fabellofibular ligament, are difficult to identify in formalin-preserved knees, which were used in this study.

Watanabe et al[31] observed that the fabellofibular ligament coursed between the fibula and the fabella and was under the greatest tension when the knee was in full extension and relaxed as the knee flexed. They postulated that the fabellofibular ligament was a major supporting structure of the posterolateral aspect of the knee.

To summarize the literature on the fabellofibular ligament, it has been described to be the structure that coursed from the tip of the fibular styloid to the region of a bony or cartilaginous fabella.[4,15,16,31,34,56,57] It appears that it may be more prominent when a bony fabella is present[4,15,16] and is under tension only when the knee is close to full extension.[4,31] In the absence of a bony fabella, the structure has also been named by some authors as the short lateral ligament.[4,15]

◆ The Arcuate Ligament: A Separate Ligament? Fact or Fiction?

It can be said without controversy that the main confusion in the literature and in clinical practice relating to posterolateral knee anatomy lies with the structures that course from the medial aspect of the fibular head and styloid to the posterolateral aspect of the knee. In the past, these structures were commonly grouped together and called the "arcuate ligament." Part of this confusion comes from the fact that individual descriptions of the arcuate, or "arched," ligament differ significantly from one another in the literature. In a statement that still holds true today, Last[14] stated over 50 years ago that the greatest confusion about posterolateral knee anatomy was in the inconsistent anatomic description of the arcuate ligament.

Dujarier[57] reported that the anterior fibers of the fibular portion of the arcuate ligament formed the short external lateral ligament. This structure was noted to course from the fibular styloid to the fabella. He was referring to the fabellofibular ligament, based on his description of this portion of the arcuate ligament.

Last[18] provided one of the first modern accounts of the arcuate ligament. In his description, he attempted to provide a more detailed account of the anatomy of some of the individual structures of the knee joint compared with anatomic textbooks at that time. Last reported that the arcuate ligament consisted of the free posterior border of the "short external lateral ligament" of old terminology (and he did not provide any reference to other articles that used old terminology). He noted that this structure had no name in the current terminology that was being revised at that time and that was subsequently developed into the *Nomina Anatomica* in 1956. From its lateral attachment on the medial aspect of the fibular head and styloid, the free posterior border of the short external lateral ligament was noted to lie over the popliteus fascia and adhere firmly to it. This would appear to be the popliteofibular ligament based upon his description (**Fig. 2–13**). Last also noted that it attached at its upper proximal end to the posterior arch of the lateral meniscus, which would be the popliteal aponeurosis to the lateral meniscus.

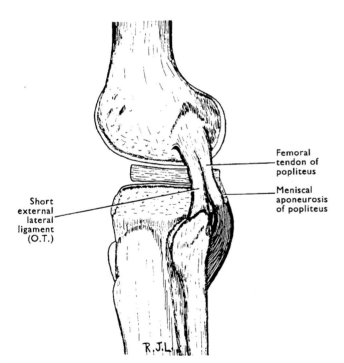

Femoral tendon of popliteus

Meniscal aponeurosis of popliteus

Short external lateral ligament (O.T.)

Figure 2–13   The lateral aspect of the left knee demonstrating the popliteus tendon and short external lateral ligament (popliteofibular ligament) of the knee. (From Last RJ. The popliteus muscle and the lateral meniscus: with a note on the attachment of the medial meniscus. J Bone Joint Surg 1950;32B:93–99, with permission.)

Last's description of the arcuate ligament would encompass both the popliteofibular ligament and the popliteal aponeurosis to the lateral meniscus, but did not include the fabellofibular ligament or the capsular arm of the short head of the biceps femoris.

Last[14] also reported that a substantial portion of the popliteus muscle arose not from the popliteus tendon but from the arcuate ligament itself. In this description, he was referring to the popliteus muscle fibers that course almost vertically in line from the popliteus complex to the lateral meniscus, which we now call the popliteal aponeurosis of the lateral meniscus. In Last's description, this comprised a portion of the arcuate ligament. In addition, Last also reported that the short external lateral ligament coursed from the fibular styloid to the region of the lateral epicondyle. Although not clearly describing which structure this may have been, it appears from an illustration (**Fig. 2–12**) that he was also referring to a portion of the popliteofibular ligament.

The follow-up article by Last[14] further described the confusion about which structures comprised the arcuate ligament. He reported that some textbooks at that time reported that the arcuate ligament arched from the fibular styloid, over the popliteus muscle, and blended with the oblique popliteal ligament. Last noted that some textbooks also appeared to demonstrate that the arcuate ligament extended from the lateral femoral condyle and posterior capsule in a triangular sheet, which attached on the fibular styloid. Last reported that two limbs were described consistently as a portion of this triangular tissue sheet that coursed off the fibular styloid. The lateral limb was dense and strong and coursed from the fibular styloid to the popliteus tendon. This would be the popliteofibular ligament. Last reported that the popliteus tendon itself was firmly attached along its lateral surface to the joint capsule and the stronger lateral limb of the arcuate ligament. This would appear to be the popliteofibular ligament and the capsular arm of the short head of the biceps femoris. The weaker medial limb of the arcuate ligament was described to curve over the popliteus muscle and attached proximally to the posterior horn of the lateral meniscus and posterior joint capsule. This would appear to be the popliteal aponeurosis to the lateral meniscus (**Fig. 2–14**).

Last[14] also reported that the upper end of the "short external lateral ligament" of old terminology was fused to the popliteus tendon near its femoral attachment, whereas the lower end diverged from the popliteus tendon to insert on the fibular styloid and medial border of the fibular head. This would appear to be the popliteofibular ligament. Last noted that the "short external lateral ligament" blended with the capsule, which attached to the popliteus tendon and was a thickened part of the posterior tibiofibular joint capsule in this area. It would appear from his article that he was referring to the popliteofibular ligament and the lateral aspect of the popliteus tendon.

Although Kaplan[20] provided an illustration of the arcuate ligament in one of his papers, he provided no description of it to supplement the illustration in this particular text. The illustration appears to show that the arcuate ligament in his description constitutes the oblique popliteal ligament medially and the capsular arm of the short head of the biceps femoris on its lateral aspect. His illustration also demonstrates that the arcuate ligament (which appears to be the fabellofibular ligament and the capsular arm of the short head of the biceps

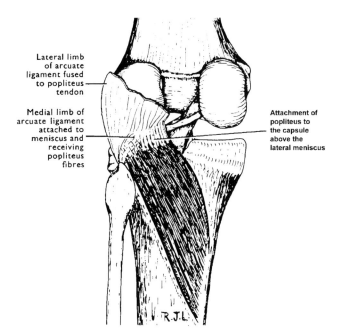

Lateral limb of arcuate ligament fused to popliteus tendon

Medial limb of arcuate ligament attached to meniscus and receiving popliteus fibres

Attachment of popliteus to the capsule above the lateral meniscus

Figure 2–14   The posterior aspect of a left knee demonstrating Last's description of the medial (popliteal aponeurosis to the lateral meniscus) and lateral limbs (popliteofibular ligament, and capsular arm of the short head of the biceps femoris) of the arcuate ligament. (From Last RJ. The popliteus muscle and the lateral meniscus: with a note on the attachment of the medial meniscus. J Bone Joint Surg 1950;32B:93–99, with permission.)

femoris) passes posterior to the inferior lateral genicular artery in his nomenclature. I should note that this relationship to the course of the inferior lateral genicular artery is important in comparing these structures in different references and will be covered in the next section (**Fig. 2–15**).

In a follow-up paper, Kaplan,[4] reported on the anatomy of the fabellofibular ligament and the short lateral ligament of the knee. He noted that previous authors' descriptions of the short lateral ligament varied somewhat, but they were similar in their text. Weitbrecht,[56] Dujarier,[57] and Vallois[34] described the proximal end of the short lateral ligament to originate at the fabella, although Last[14,18] had placed the proximal attachment at the popliteus tendon near its femoral attachment. In all cases, the distal attachment of the short lateral ligament was noted to be to the fibular styloid. Kaplan noted that the short lateral ligament had been described as a part of the "lateral arch" of the arcuate ligament or as a reinforcement of the posterior capsule. Kaplan noted that these descriptions of the short lateral ligament were primarily consistent with what he termed the fabellofibular ligament.

To further understand the fabellofibular ligament–short lateral ligament complex, Kaplan,[4] also performed numerous comparative anatomy and human knee dissections. He noted that the medial arch of the arcuate ligament was formed by the lateral border of the oblique popliteal ligament as it arched over the popliteus muscle. Kaplan's observations about the lateral arch of the

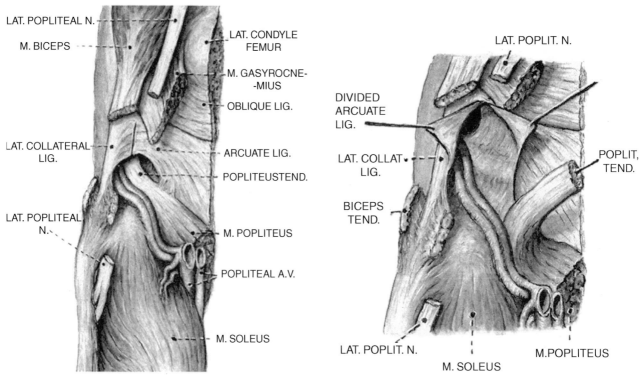

Figure 2–15 The posterior view of the left knee demonstrating the relationship between the lateral collateral ligament (fibular collateral ligament), popliteus tendon, and inferior lateral genicular vessels. There does not appear to be a popliteofibular ligament or a related structure in this illustration. (From Kaplan EB. Surgical approach to the lateral (peroneal) side of the knee joint. Surg Gynecol Obstet 1957;104:346–356, with permission.)

arcuate ligament were written in a narrative style, which allows us to compare his dissections to our current understanding of the anatomy of the individual structures of the posterolateral aspect of the knee. Kaplan noted that some fibers of the lateral arch of the arcuate ligament ran from the fibula and frequently blended with the posterior capsule of the proximal tibiofibular joint to such an extent that it could not easily be dissected from the capsule or the fascia covering the popliteus muscle. Both his description and his accompanying illustration demonstrate that the structure that he referred to was the popliteofibular ligament. A further support of my interpretation of this is that he mentioned that the inferior lateral genicular artery passed posterior to the postero-proximal tibiofibular joint capsule and the lateral arch of the arcuate ligament (or the popliteofibular ligament) **(Fig. 2–16)**. Kaplan also noted that the inferior lateral genicular artery ran between the lateral arch of the arcuate ligament (the popliteofibular ligament) and the short lateral (fabellofibular) ligament. He reported that the lateral arch of the arcuate ligament provided an additional reinforcement of the posterior capsule of the knee joint where the popliteus muscle attached to the coronary ligament of the lateral meniscus (the popliteal aponeurosis to the lateral meniscus). He also noted that the lateral arch of the arcuate ligament was adherent to the posterior tibiofibular capsule at the

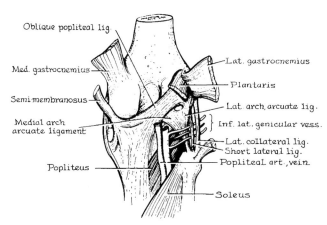

Figure 2–16 Posterior view of a right knee. The inferior lateral genicular vessels are seen coursing between the arcuate ligament (popliteofibular ligament) and the short lateral ligament (fabellofibular ligament and capsular arm of the short head of the biceps femoris) in Kaplan's description of this anatomy. (From Kaplan EB. The fabellofibular and short lateral ligaments of the knee joint. J Bone Joint Surg 1961;43A:169–179, with permission.)

popliteus musculotendinous junction. This structure definitely appears to be the popliteofibular ligament. Kaplan also noted that the medial border of the fabellofibular ligament blended with the lateral arch of the arcuate ligament. This would appear to be the capsular arm of the short head of the biceps femoris and the popliteofibular ligament respectively.

Lovejoy and Harden[26] reported that in their dissections of 15 cadaveric knees, they found attachments of the popliteus tendon to the femur and an attachment to the fibula in all knees, which along with a base that attached to the posterior capsule and meniscus (the popliteal aponeurosis to the lateral meniscus), formed a Y-shaped ligament. They stated that previous descriptions of an arcuate ligament actually were describing this Y-shaped ligament of the popliteus complex structure (which was formed by the popliteus tendon, popliteofibular ligament, and popliteal aponeurosis to the lateral meniscus). They stated that the view that the arcuate ligament was a separate and distinct structure with attachments to the fibula, popliteus, and posterior knee joint was distorted and not supported at all by their finding. They noted that the arcuate ligament was not a distinct structure, but was actually a condensation of fibers that originated from the popliteus. Unfortunately, their work was in the anatomy literature rather than the orthopaedic literature so it was not well noted or recognized.

Hughston et al[45] reported that the posterolateral part of the knee formed a single "full functional unit," which they called the "arcuate complex." The arcuate complex was noted to be formed by the fibular collateral ligament, arcuate ligament, and the tendoaponeurotic portion of the popliteus muscle. Hughston et al's description of an arcuate complex referred to the structures that attached to the fibular head and styloid. I was fortunate enough to have reviewed many of Hughston's operative notes and data recording forms during my fellowship year training in 1993–1994. Dr. Hughston drew an illustration with colored pencils of the findings of every surgery that he performed. It was clear from my review of his drawings that my current work and attempts to build a common nomenclature is a further step along from his outstanding original work. Unfortunately, many physicians were confused by the lumping together of these structures with the arcuate complex.

Seebacher et al[15] also reported on the structure of the arcuate ligament, as they knew it at that point in time, in their description of the three layers of the posterolateral aspect of the knee. Their deepest layer (layer III), reported to be part of the lateral capsule, was described as occurring in two laminae. The superficial lamina was described as encompassing the fibular collateral ligament and ended posteriorly at the fabellofibular ligament or short lateral ligament. This would appear to be the lateral aponeurosis of the long and short heads of the biceps femoris, which ended at the capsular arm of the short head of the biceps femoris. The deeper part of the "posterolateral part of the capsule" was noted to form both the coronary ligament to the lateral meniscus and the hiatus to the popliteus tendon (i.e., the popliteomeniscal fascicles). The deep (inner) lamina was described to terminate posteriorly as the "Y-shaped arcuate ligament." They reported that the arcuate ligament spanned the junction from the popliteus muscle and tendon (i.e., at its musculotendinous junction) to the fibula. Their description of the arcuate ligament fits the current description of the popliteofibular ligament. In addition to this description, they also stated that the arcuate ligament had a vertical limb that coursed from the fibula to the condylar plate (the fabella region). They also described a medial fanning of the arcuate ligament where it joined the fibers of the oblique popliteal ligament. Because they only briefly mentioned this vertical limb of the arcuate ligament, and it does not fit their descriptions or illustrations of the arcuate ligament in the rest of the article, it appears they were also describing the fabellofibular ligament (and along with it the capsular arm of the short head of the biceps femoris) to be a portion of the arcuate ligament in a part of the description of their dissections. The two capsular laminae (i.e., the fabellofibular and capsular arm of the short head of the biceps femoris and popliteofibular ligaments, respectively, of the superficial and deep laminae) were always noted to be separated from each other by the inferior lateral genicular artery, in the region where both structures attached at the apex of the fibular styloid (**Fig. 2–17**). Although Seebacher et al[15] found three different variations of the size of the superficial and deep laminae of their descriptions, they noted that at all times a reinforcing structure of variable size was present that coursed from the fibula to the musculotendinous junction of the popliteus. We now know this to be the popliteofibular ligament.

Müller[53] reported that the arcuate ligament complex consisted of the fabellofibular ligament of Vallois,[34] the deep portions of the posterolateral capsule, and the meniscotibial attachments. It was noted that the most proximal portion of the arcuate ligament was at the fabella. His descriptions and illustrations of the arcuate (popliteal) ligament appear to show that it was composed of the popliteofibular ligament, the popliteal aponeurosis of the lateral meniscus, and the capsular arm of the short head of the biceps femoris. Although the fabellofibular ligament was noted to be part of the arcuate ligament complex, it was illustrated as a separate structure in his work.

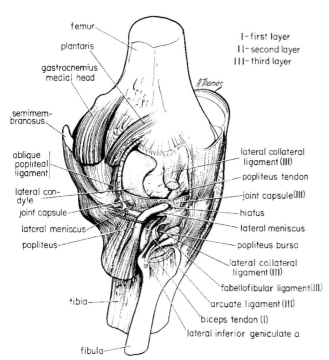

femur
plantaris
gastrocnemius
medial head

I - first layer
II - second layer
III - third layer

semimem-
branosus

oblique
popliteal
ligament

lateral con-
dyle

joint capsule

lateral meniscus

popliteus

lateral collateral
ligament (III)

popliteus tendon

joint capsule (III)

hiatus

lateral meniscus

popliteus bursa

lateral collateral
ligament (III)

fabellofibular ligament (III)

tibia

arcuate ligament (III)

biceps tendon (I)

lateral inferior geniculate a.

fibula

Figure 2–17 The posterolateral aspect of a right knee. The arcuate ligament (popliteofibular ligament) was noted to course between the fibular head and the popliteus. It was also deep (anterior) to the inferior lateral genicular artery. (From Seebacher JR, Inglis AE, Marshall JL, Warren RF. The structure of the posterolateral aspect of the knee. J Bone Joint Surg 1982;64A:536–541, with permission.)

Sudasna and Harnsiriwattanagit[16] noted that it was very difficult to interpret the findings of previous studies of posterolateral knee anatomy because of the confusion related to the terms used to describe them. They felt that this was particularly true for the arcuate ligament, short lateral ligament, and the fabellofibular ligament. In their dissection of formalin-preserved cadavers, they identified an arcuate ligament in 24% of the knees. In their description of the arcuate ligament, they noted it to be thin and membranous, with fibers adherent to the superficial surface of the posterior aspect of the popliteus tendon in most cases. They felt the arcuate ligament was weak, and theorized it could not play a role as an important static stabilizer of the knee. In their one anatomic dissection picture, their arcuate ligament appears to be equivalent to the capsular arm of the short head of the biceps femoris[38] in that it was a broad-based sheet of fascial tissue that coursed from the tip of the fibular styloid to the posterolateral capsule of the knee toward the region of the fabella or a cartilaginous fabella analogue and lateral gastrocnemius tendon. One point of confusion in their article is that in their conclusions, they note that the inferior lateral genicular artery coursed between the arcuate ligament (which in their description appears to be the capsular arm of the short head of the short head of the biceps femoris) and the fabellofibular ligament. Nowhere else in their manuscript is

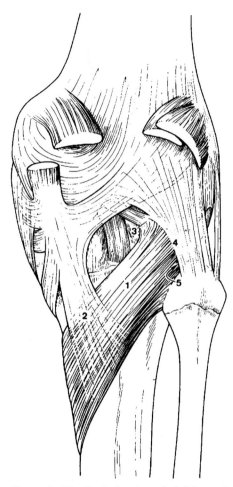

Figure 2–18   Posterior view of a left knee. 1, popliteus muscle; 2, distal semimembranosus expansion; 3, posteosuperior popliterosuperior fascicle; 4, arcuate ligament; 5, popliteofibular ligament. The "arcuate popliteal" ligament[7] (capsular arm of the short head of the biceps femoris and fabellofibular ligament) is noted to course from the top of the fibular styloid to the posterolateral capsule and oblique popliteal ligament. (From Stäubli HU, Birrer S. The popliteus tendon and its fascicles at the popliteus hiatus: gross anatomy and functional arthroscopic evaluation with and without anterior cruciate ligament deficiency. Arthroscopy 1990;6:209–220, with permission.)

this described or illustrated, but we have found the inferior lateral genicular artery to be deeper (anterior) to both of their described structures and posterior only to the popliteofibular ligament at this region of the knee.

Stäubli and Birrer[22] illustrated the "arcuate popliteal" ligament in their article. No text was written to describe their illustration of this structure in their work. Based on this illustration, it appears that they were referring to the fabellofibular ligament and capsular arm of the short head of the biceps femoris as constituting the "arcuate popliteal" ligament (**Fig. 2–18**). Later in their article, they correlated their studies to the study of Seebacher et al,[15] and reported that Seebacher et al's description of the deep lamina of layer III (which Seebacher et al called the arcuate ligament), which coursed between the popliteus musculotendinous junction and the fibula, coincided with Stäubli and Birrer's description of the anterior and posterior limbs of the popliteofibular ligament.

In a separate article, Stäubli and Rauschning[25] also further reported on the anatomy of the arcuate popliteal ligament. They reported that the arcuate popliteal ligament joined with the lateral aspect of the popliteus muscle and that the inferior lateral genicular artery ran deep (anterior) to it. In this regard, little description of this structure was given in their text. However, in reviewing their illustration and figure legend, one can see that this structure courses from the tip of the fibular styloid and runs to the posterolateral joint capsule and oblique popliteal ligament (i.e., the region of the fabella). It would therefore appear that they were referring to the arcuate popliteal ligament as a portion of the fabellofibular ligament and the capsular arm of the short head of the biceps femoris. In summarizing Stäubli and coauthors' works,[22,25] it is clear that they were referring to a different structure as the arcuate ligament from previous authors' descriptions that primarily appeared to describe the arcuate ligament as the popliteofibular ligament.

Hughston[58] noted that the arcuate ligament blended with the oblique popliteal ligament, popliteus fascia, and other surrounding fascial layers and had a distal attachment to the fibula, tibia, and meniscus. He postulated that each of the ligaments in the arcuate complex, except for the popliteus tendon, could be considered to be an aponeurosis of the long and short heads of the biceps femoris (the capsular arm of the short head of the biceps femoris) and the central portion of the popliteus muscle (the popliteal aponeurosis of the lateral meniscus). Hughston also noted that the arcuate ligament (which appears to be the popliteofibular ligament and was different from the arcuate complex) meshed with the meniscotibial ligament, which attached to the popliteus muscle (i.e., the anteroinferior popliteomeniscal fascicle), as it coursed from the fibular head. The more medial portion of the popliteus muscle was felt to form the aponeurosis of the "tibial portion of the arcuate ligament" (the popliteal aponeurosis to the lateral meniscus). Hughston also noted that fibrous tissues from the lateral gastrocnemius tendon meshed into the arcuate ligament fibers. We now believe this is the capsular arm of the short head of the biceps femoris.

Watanabe et al[31] noted that the three main posterolateral knee structures were the arcuate ligament, fabellofibular ligament, and the popliteus muscle with origin from the fibular head (i.e., the popliteofibular ligament) (**Fig. 2–19**). They stated that the arcuate ligament was posterior to the inferior lateral genicular artery. They noted that the arcuate ligament was a thin triangular band of capsular fibers, which originated at the posterior aspect of the fibula, and arched upward and medially over the popliteus tendon with no strong connection from this triangular band of fibers to the popliteus tendon seen. They noted that the popliteal origin from the fibular head (popliteofibular ligament) was distinct and deeper than the arcuate ligament. The popliteofibular ligament was noted to be a distinct condensation of fibers that coursed from the fibular head to the posterior fibers of the popliteus tendon, which blended into the proximal posterior tibiofibular joint capsule. They postulated that the arcuate ligament in their dissections was too thin to act as a restraint to posterolateral rotation. It would appear that their arcuate ligament description was what we

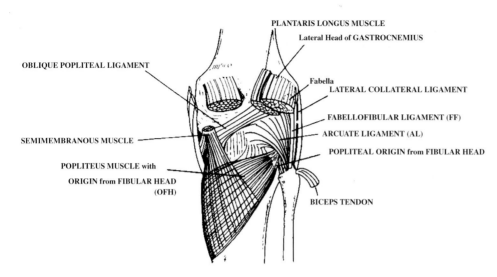

PLANTARIS LONGUS MUSCLE

Lateral Head of GASTROCNEMIUS

OBLIQUE POPLITEAL LIGAMENT

Fabella

LATERAL COLLATERAL LIGAMENT

FABELLOFIBULAR LIGAMENT (FF)

ARCUATE LIGAMENT (AL)

SEMIMEMBRANOUS MUSCLE

POPLITEAL ORIGIN from FIBULAR HEAD

POPLITEUS MUSCLE with

ORIGIN from FIBULAR HEAD

(OFH)

BICEPS TENDON

Figure 2–19 Posterior view of the right knee. The fabellofibular ligament, arcuate ligament (capsular arm of the short head of the biceps femoris), and popliteal origin from the fibular head (popliteofibular ligament), according to Watanabe's dissections. (From Watanabe Y, Moriya H, Takahashi K, et al. Functional anatomy of the posterolateral structures of the knee. Arthroscopy 1993;9:57–62, with permission.)

refer to currently as the capsular arm of the short head of the biceps femoris. It should also be noted that their dissections were performed on formalin-preserved cadaveric, rather than fresh-frozen knees, which can often be more difficult to flex and extend and define fine tissue planes during the dissection process.

Maynard et al[29] discussed the "rediscovery" of the popliteofibular ligament in their award-winning paper that they presented at the American Orthopaedic Society for Sports Medicine Annual Meeting in 1994. In addition to their description of the anatomy of the popliteofibular ligament, they also described the anatomy of the arcuate ligament. They noted that the fibers of the arcuate ligament originated on the fibular head, superficial (posterior) to the popliteofibular ligament attachment, and coursed medially off the fibular head and blended with the oblique popliteal ligament fibers. It would appear that they were referring to the capsular arm of the short head of the biceps femoris. Maynard et al noted that they could distinguish the difference between the arcuate ligament and the popliteofibular ligament by the orientation of their fibers. No further descriptions or illustrations were provided, but it appears that their description of the arcuate ligament was the capsular arm of the short head of the biceps femoris. In addition, they noted that their description of the arcuate ligament differed from previous articles' descriptions of it from their research center.[15,32]

To summarize the literature on the description of the arcuate ligament, it is clear that varying authors have called different structures the arcuate ligament. To understand this varying anatomy, an attempt has been made to decipher their descriptions based on the author's text, illustrations, and anatomic landmarks, especially the structures' relationship to the inferior lateral genicular artery. In general, the earlier authors who were reviewed here tended to have more qualitative descriptions rather than a detailed analysis of the structures.

It would appear that some authors were referring to the popliteofibular ligament as constituting all or a majority of the arcuate ligament.[4,14,15,18,53] In addition, the popliteal aponeurosis to the lateral meniscus has also been described as part of the arcuate ligament.[4,14,18,58] In fact, Lovejoy and Harden[26] reported that the arcuate ligament was not a distinct structure, but rather a Y-shaped condensation formed by the popliteus tendon, popliteofibular ligament, and the popliteal aponeurosis to the lateral meniscus.

However, other authors' descriptions of the arcuate ligament described it as a combination of the fabellofibular ligament, or its homologue, the short lateral ligament, and the capsular arm of the short head of the biceps femoris.[16,20,22,25,29,31] In this description of the arcuate ligament, Kaplan[4,20] and Stäubli and Rauschning[25] noted that the medial fibers, or limb, of the arcuate ligament included the fibers of the oblique popliteal ligament. The medial limb, or arch, of the arcuate ligament has also been described to be the popliteal aponeurosis to the lateral meniscus[14] as well as the oblique popliteal ligament.[4,15,29]

From this overview of the literature, it would appear that those authors who recognized the presence of the popliteofibular ligament reported that the arcuate ligament was primarily composed of what is now recognized as the fabellofibular ligament and the capsular arm of the short head of the biceps femoris,[4,16,20,22,25,29,31] whereas those authors who did not recognize the presence of the popliteofibular ligament usually called it the arcuate ligament.[14,15,18,53] The only exception to this observation was Kaplan, who noted the presence of the popliteofibular ligament in some studies,[20,23,24] but also described it as a lateral arch of the arcuate ligament in another study.[4] In any event, it does appear that the arcuate ligament is not a distinct separate structure. In that regard, due to the confusion that it has created about the anatomy of the posterolateral knee, I recommend that the term *arcuate ligament* be dropped to avoid further confusion as to which structure it represents.

◆ Inferior Lateral Genicular Artery

The inferior lateral genicular artery is an important landmark to use in comparing differences in the literature on individual structures at the posterolateral aspect of the knee in the region of the fibular head and styloid. Kaplan[4] reported that the inferior lateral genicular artery crossed the joint capsule anterior to the "lateral arch" of the arcuate ligament. He was referring to the fabellofibular ligament and capsular arm of the short head of the biceps femoris. Seebacher et al[15] reported that the superficial and deep laminae (i.e., the fabellofibular ligament and popliteofibular ligament, respectively) of layer III of their three-layer description of posterolateral knee anatomy were separated from each other by this artery. Sudasna and Harnsiriwattanagit[16] noted in their conclusions that the inferior lateral genicular artery coursed between the arcuate ligament (i.e., the capsular arm of the short head of the biceps femoris) and the fabellofibular ligament. It was not described or illustrated elsewhere in their paper. Stäubli and coauthors[22,25] also reported that the inferior lateral genicular artery was anterior (deep) to the "arcuate popliteal" ligament (fabellofibular ligament and capsular arm of the short head of the biceps femoris) and posterior (superficial) to the popliteofibular ligament. Watanabe[31] also stated that the arcuate ligament (i.e., the capsular arm of the short head of the biceps femoris) was posterior to the inferior lateral genicular artery.

To summarize the literature on the inferior lateral genicular artery, it has been demonstrated to course between the structure that courses from the fibula to the popliteus musculotendinous junction (the popliteofibular ligament) and the other structure that courses from the fibula to the fabella or fabella region (fabellofibular ligament).[4,15,22,25,31] Only in Sudansa and Harnsiriwattanagit's[16] work was this artery reported to course differently. Therefore, the inferior lateral genicular artery has been found to be an important landmark to compare the results of differing authors in their conflicting nomenclature for the structures that coursed from the fibular head and styloid and attached to the structures over the posterolateral aspect of the knee.

◆ Conclusions

A review of the historical literature regarding the anatomy of the posterolateral knee demonstrates why it is useful in understanding the anatomy of posterolateral knee, but also at times why it is confusing and conflicting. The varying nomenclature among different authors has made it difficult to compare studies. In addition, as time has gone on, there has been more of a tendency to name individual anatomic structures rather than to identify structures according to layers of the knee.[8,15,35] The layered approach to describe structures, or groups of structures, is very difficult to remember, understand, and teach without hands-on dissection experiences. It has also been observed that these individual anatomic structures have been present in virtually all knees and that the wide variation in the incidence of specific individual structures has been based on the variable understanding among research centers of the anatomy of the posterolateral knee and differences in their respective dissection techniques, and not in an actual true variation in the incidence of these structures.

It appears that the major confusion about posterolateral knee anatomy found in the orthopaedic literature lies with the structures that course from the fibular head and styloid and attach to the popliteus complex and joint capsule over the posterolateral aspect of the knee. In the past, these structures, or a portion of these structures, were grouped together and called the "arcuate," or arched, ligament. This is because those structures that attach to the fibular head and course to the posterolateral aspect of the knee form an arched-like appearance, in their continuity with the oblique popliteal ligament medially, over the posterior aspect of the knee. The inferior lateral genicular artery has been found to be an important landmark to compare descriptions of these structures in different studies, and previous authors' descriptions, to allow identification of the structures described between these different studies. The popliteofibular ligament is anterior to the inferior lateral genicular artery. The popliteofibular ligament is the only structure that is anterior to the inferior lateral genicular artery where it crosses at the posterior aspect of the fibular styloid. Therefore, the arcuate ligament of Seebacher et al's[15] study was in actuality the popliteofibular ligament, based on their description and their illustration of its location relative to the inferior lateral genicular artery. The fabellofibular ligament courses from its attachment just lateral to the tip of the fibular styloid to its attachment in the region of a fabella or a fabella (cartilaginous) analogue. The fabellofibular ligament is posterior to the inferior lateral genicular artery. The large capsular expansion that courses from the tip of the fibular styloid to the posterolateral capsule and lateral gastrocnemius tendon is the capsular arm of the short head of the biceps femoris and its distal border is the fabellofibular ligament.[39] It appears that this structure is what has also been called the lateral arch of the arcuate ligament in other studies.[4]

The short (external) lateral ligament of some studies[4,15,34,56,57] appears to be the fabellofibular ligament, and one author has tied these two structures together as being the same structure.[4] Another author[18] reported that the short external lateral ligament was the arcuate ligament, and his text clearly demonstrates that he was referring to the popliteofibular ligament. The difference in nomenclature for these different posterolateral knee structures has been a main source of confusion in the literature.

Although it is recognized that varying nomenclature may appear in the orthopaedic literature based on one's training and the region of the world in which studies are performed, it is also desirable that a standard terminology be developed so that anatomic comparisons, biomechanical studies, magnetic resonance imaging scans, and surgical reconstructions can be compared more easily. It is also important to obtain a standard nomenclature for purposes of instruction for standard anatomy, radiographic imaging, and surgical repairs. I recommend that the terminology used in Chapter 3 on the specific anatomic structures of the posterolateral knee serve as a building block of standard nomenclature for the anatomic structures of the posterolateral aspect of the knee.

References

1. Fürst CM. Der Musculus Popliteus und Seine Sehne. In: Ueber ihre Entwicklung und uber Einige Damit Zusammenhangende Bildungen. Lunds Universitets Arsskrift Band 39. Lund, Germany: E. Malstroms Buchdruckerei, 1903 (German)
2. Taylor G, Bonney V. On the homology and morphology of the popliteus muscle: a contribution to comparative myology. J Anat Physiol 1905;40:34–50
3. Herzmark MH. The evolution of the knee joint. J Bone Joint Surg 1938;20:77–84
4. Kaplan EB. The fabellofibular and short lateral ligaments of the knee joint. J Bone Joint Surg 1961;43A:169–179
5. Fabbriciani C, Oransky M, Zoppi U. The popliteal muscle: an anatomical study. Arch Ital Anat Embriol 1982;87:203–217
6. Haines RW. The tetrapod knee joint. J Anat 1942;76:270–301
7. Kaplan EB. The iliotibial tract. Clinical and morphological significance. J Bone Joint Surg 1958;40A:817–832
8. Marshall JL, Girgis FG, Zelko RR. The biceps femoris tendon and its functional significance. J Bone Joint Surg 1972;54A:1444–1450
9. Maissiat JH. Etudes de Physique Animale. Paris: Bethune et Plon, 1843 (French)
10. Jakob RP, Hassler H, Stäubli HU. Observations on rotatory instability of the lateral compartment of the knee: experimental studies on the functional anatomy and pathomechanism of the true and reversed pivot shift sign. Acta Orthop Scand Suppl 1981;191:1–32

11. LaPrade RF. The medial collateral ligament complex and posterolateral aspect of the knee. In: Sports Medicine Orthopaedic Knowledge Update (OKU). Chicago: American Academy of Orthopaedic Surgeons, 1999

12. Thompson WO, Thaete FL, Fu FH, Dye SF. Tibial meniscal dynamics using three-dimensional reconstruction of magnetic resonance images. Am J Sports Med 1991;19:210–216

13. Nomina Anatomica (Paris). Revised by the International Congress of Anatomists. Baltimore, MD: Williams and Wilkins, 1956

14. Last RJ. The popliteus muscle and the lateral meniscus: with a note on the attachment of the medial meniscus. J Bone Joint Surg 1950;32B:93–99

15. Seebacher JR, Inglis AE, Marshall JL, Warren RF. The structure of the posterolateral aspect of the knee. J Bone Joint Surg 1982;64A:536–541

16. Sudasna S, Harnsiriwattanagit K. The ligamentous structures of the posterolateral aspect of the knee. Bull Hosp Joint Dis 1990;50:35–40

17. Sutton JB. On the nature of certain ligaments. J Anat Physiol 1884;18:225–238

18. Last RJ. Some anatomical details of the knee joint. J Bone Joint Surg 1948;30B: 683–688

19. Gray DJ, Gardner E. Prenatal development of the human knee and superior tibiofibular joints. Am J Anat 1950;86:235–287

20. Kaplan EB. Surgical approach to the lateral (peroneal) side of the knee joint. Surg Gynecol Obstet 1957;104:346–356

21. Higgins H. The popliteus muscle. J Anat 1894;29:569–573

22. Stäubli HU, Birrer S. The popliteus tendon and its fascicles at the popliteus hiatus: gross anatomy and functional arthroscopic evaluation with and without anterior cruciate ligament deficiency. Arthroscopy 1990;6:209–220

23. Kaplan EB. Factors responsible for the stability of the knee joint. Bull Hosp Joint Dis 1957B;18:51–59

24. Kaplan EB. Some aspects of functional anatomy of the human knee joint. Clin Orthop 1962;23:18–29

25. Stäubli HU, Rauschning W. Popliteus tendon and lateral meniscus: gross and multiplanar cryosectional anatomy of the knee. Am J Knee Surg 1991;4:110–121

26. Lovejoy JF, Harden TT. Popliteus muscle in man. Anat Rec 1971;169:727–730

27. Reis FP, Ferraz de Carvalho CA. Anatomical study on the proximal attachments of the human popliteus muscle. Rev Bras de Pesq Med e Biol 1975;8:373–380

28. Cohn AK, Mains DB. Popliteal hiatus of the lateral meniscus. Am J Sports Med 1979;7:221–226

29. Maynard MJ, Deng X-H, Wickiewicz TL, Warren RF. The popliteofibular ligament: rediscovery of a key element in posterolateral instability. Am J Sports Med 1996;24:311–316

30. Oransky M, Canero G, Maiotti M. Embryonic development of the posterolateral structures of the knee. Anat Rec 1989;225:347–354

31. Watanabe Y, Moriya H, Takahashi K, et al. Functional anatomy of the posterolateral structures of the knee. Arthroscopy 1993;9:57–62

32. Gollehon DL, Torzilli PA, Warren RF. The role of the posterolateral and cruciate ligaments in the stability of the human knee: a biomechanical study. J Bone Joint Surg 1987;69A:233–242

33. Sussman PS, Simonian PT, Wickiewicz TL, Warren RF. Development of the popliteomeniscal fasciculi in the human knee joint. Arthroscopy 2001;17:14–18

34. Vallois HV. Etudes Anatomiques de l'Articulation du Genou Ches les Primates. Thesis, Universite de Montpellier, No. 63, 1914 (French)

35. Sneath RS. The insertion of the biceps femoris. J Anat 1955;89:550–553
36. Kaplan EB. Comparative anatomy of the extensor digitorum longus in relation to the knee joint. Anat Rec 1958B;131:129–149
37. LaPrade RF, Hamilton CD. The fibular collateral ligament–biceps femoris bursa: an anatomic study. Am J Sports Med 1997;25:439–443
38. Terry GC, LaPrade RF. The biceps femoris muscle complex at the knee: its anatomy and injury patterns associated with acute anterolateral-anteromedial rotatory instability. Am J Sports Med 1996;24:2–8
39. Terry GC, LaPrade RF. The posterolateral aspect of the knee: anatomy and surgical approach. Am J Sports Med 1996;24:732–739
40. Terry GC, Hughston JC, Norwood LA. The anatomy of the iliopatellar band and iliotibial tract. Am J Sports Med 1986;14:39–45
41. Lobenhoffer P, Posel P, Witt S, Piehler J, Wirth CJ. Distal femoral fixation of the iliotibial tract. Arch Orthop Trauma Surg 1987;106:285–290
42. Gerdy PN. Troisier Monographic Maladies des Organes du Mouvement OS Muscles. Paris: Chez Victor Masson, 1855 (French)
43. Segond P. Recherches cliniques et experimentales sur les epanchcments sanguins du genou par entorse. Progress Med 1879;VII:1–84 (French)
44. Johnson LL. Lateral capsular ligament complex: anatomical and surgical considerations. Am J Sports Med 1979;7:156–160
45. Hughston JC, Andrews JR, Cross MJ, Moschi A. Classification of knee ligament instabilities. Part II: the lateral compartment. J Bone Joint Surg 1976;58A:173–179
46. Winslow JB. An Anatomical Exposition of the Structure of the Human Body. London, 1733
47. Soames RW, ed. Skeletal system. In: Gray's Anatomy. New York: Churchill-Livingstone, 1995:703
48. Poirier P, Charpy A. Traite d'Anatomie Humaine 1901;2:238–241 (French)
49. Cave AEJ, Porteous CJ. The attachments of the semimembranosus. Proc Anat Soc Gr Brit Ire 1957;41:638
50. Cave AEJ, Porteous CJ. A note on the semimembranosus muscle. Ann R Coll Surg Eng 1959;24:251–256
51. Cross MJ. The functional significance of the distal attachment of the semimembranosus muscle in man. J Anat 1974;118:401
52. Warren LF, Marshall JL. The supporting structures of the layers on the medial side of the knee: an anatomical analysis. J Bone Joint Surg 1979;61A:56–62
53. Müller W. The Knee: Form, Function and Ligament Reconstruction. New York: Springer-Verlag, 1983
54. Zivanovic S. A note on the gorilla knee joint. Anat Anz 1972;130:91–98
55. Stäubli HU. Posteromedial and posterolateral capsular injuries associated with posterior cruciate ligament insufficiency. Sports Med Arthro Rev 1994;2:146–164
56. Weitbrecht J. Syndesmologia, sive Historia Ligamentorum Corporis Humani quam Secundum Observations Anatomicas Concinnauit. Petropoli, Typographia Academiae Scientiorum, 1742 (Latin)
57. Dujarier C. Anatomie des Membres; Dissection; Anatomie Topographique. Paris: G. Steinheil, 1905 (French)
58. Hughston JC. Knee Ligaments. Injury and Repairs. Chicago: Mosby, 1993

3

Comprehensive Anatomy of the Structures of the Posterolateral Knee

It can be argued that one of the biggest sources of confusion in sports medicine is the individual anatomic structures of the posterolateral corner of the knee. Although it has been argued that this is due to multiple factors, including the reported varying incidences of occurrence of the different structures, evolutionary changes over time, and other factors, I believe that most of the problems related to understanding the posterolateral corner of the knee are due to varying dissection techniques and the resulting competing nomenclature for many of these structures. This chapter reviews the standard terminology that has been proposed in peer-reviewed publications, which is based on a consistent anatomic course and attachment pattern, the corresponding relationship to adjacent structures, and descriptions for individual anatomic structures. This review of the individual structures of the posterolateral corner of the knee can be applied in clinical practice to both diagnose injuries clinically and on MRI scans, and to perform repairs or reconstructions of these structures when patients present with pathology.

As reviewed in Chapter 2, there have been some evolutionary changes in the anatomic relationships among the fibular head, popliteus tendon, and the biceps femoris muscle that have made the anatomy of the posterolateral corner much more complex than other areas of the knee. At an earlier evolutionary time, the fibular head did articulate with the femur and it gradually migrated distally to its current position, where it articulates with the posterolateral tibial articular surface.[1-4] In addition, the popliteus muscle originated on the fibula when the fibula articulated with the femur. As the distal migration of the fibula occurred in higher order animals, the popliteus tendon over time acquired a femoral attachment that appears to be due to development of the remnant of the fibulofemoral meniscus into the popliteus tendon.[1-6] In addition, as the proximal fibula migrated distally, it appears to have pulled the lateral capsule distally with it, which, in turn, formed the popliteal hiatus.[5] Also, while the popliteus tendon obtained an attachment to the lateral aspect of the femur during the course of evolutionary development, the popliteus complex also maintained its attachment to the fibula (popliteofibular ligament).[5] Other factors that have made the anatomy of the posterolateral knee complex and somewhat unique in humans is the change in the insertion of the biceps femoris complex from the lateral capsule and proximal tibia in lower animal species and primates[7–10] to attach to the fibula and other posterolateral structures in humans. In all other animal species, the biceps femoris is the main superficial structure over the lateral aspect of the knee. It does not appear that there are any animal species that have a direct attachment of the biceps femoris to the fibula. The other factor that has made the anatomy of the posterolateral knee complex unique in humans is that it appears that only humans have an iliotibial band, which forms the main superficial covering over the anterolateral aspect of the knee.[7,11]

As reviewed in Chapter 2, the inconsistent terminology in the literature for the posterolateral knee has significantly added to clinicians' misunderstanding of posterolateral knee anatomy. For example, the "short lateral ligament" has been used to describe the fabellofibular ligament,[4,12–15] the popliteofibular ligament,[16,17] and the lateral limb of the posterior "arcuate" ligament.[18] Kaplan[4] summarized the literature and reported that the short lateral ligament and the fabellofibular ligament were homologous structures, with the short lateral ligament present when a bony fabella was absent.

Although some authors have found varying incidences of the presence of the fabellofibular ligament,[14,19] I believe that this variation was due to the lack of standard nomenclature and to differences in dissection techniques. With our definition of this structure as the distal edge of the capsular arm of the short head of the biceps femoris, and with the understanding that the fabellofibular ligament is tight in extension and becomes quite lax and hard to define with the knee flexed, we have found it to be present in all dissected knees. In addition, the structure was noted to be very difficult to identify in formalin-preserved knees because it is difficult to preserve and dissect it out, as well as because of its thin fascial substance in most knees. Although I have not quantitated it specifically in our peer-reviewed studies, the size and stoutness of the fabellofibular ligament seems to correlate with the presence and size of a bony fabella.

In spite of all these differences in nomenclature and evolutionary changes over time, however, the largest source of confusion in the literature about the posterolateral knee was the composition and presence of the "arcuate" ligament.[4,12,14–26] Although some authors have reported it to be a separate and distinct structure, I have found it not to be a separate structure, but rather a group of structures. In effect, the previous literature named several different structures located in close proximity as the arcuate ligament and as time evolved and it became recognized that the popliteofibular ligament was a distinct structure, those centers that did not recognize that the popliteofibular ligament had been called the arcuate ligament in the past were now defining it as portions of the capsular arm of the short head of the biceps femoris. Together, these separate individual structures combine to form an arched, or "arcuate," shape over the posterior aspect of the knee. I would recommend that the term *arcuate ligament* be dropped due to the confusion created in the past about which structure it refers to. The use of specific anatomic nomenclature for individual structures will help us all perform biomechanical, clinical, and radiographic studies that will lead to better surgical treatment for those patients who have posterolateral knee injuries.

In addition, I have noted a lot of difficulty in the identification of the normal attachment sites of the fibular collateral ligament, popliteus tendon, and popliteofibular ligament, which are the main static stabilizers of the posterolateral knee, at the time of acute injury or chronic repairs or reconstructions. The lack of distinct anatomic descriptions and a lack of references to bony landmarks,[1,3,5–8,14–20,23,24,26–31] led to our study of the quantitative spatial relationships and attachment sites for these particular structures.[32]

Iliotibial Band

The iliotibial band, also commonly called the iliotibial tract, is composed of four main structures. An incision over the lateral aspect of the knee exposes the large sheet of tissue that comprises the superficial layer of the iliotibial band. This superficial layer of the iliotibial band covers a large portion of the lateral aspect of the knee. The distal aspects of the iliotibial band converge to primarily attach at Gerdy's tubercle (**Fig. 3–1**).

A curvilinear anterior expansion of the superficial layer is the iliopatellar band.[33,34] The iliopatellar band courses from the main portion of the superficial layer to extend to the lateral border of the patella. The iliopatellar band is important in patellofemoral tracking, and its distal edge, which courses from the distolateral aspect of the patella down to the attachment of the iliotibial band on Gerdy's tubercle, is the lateral patellotibial ligament. In those patients who receive an overzealous lateral release and end up with symptomatic medial patellar subluxation, a reconstruction of this band can be performed[35] to stop this symptomatic iatrogenic medial patellar subluxation.

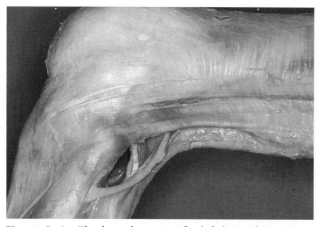

Figure 3–1   The lateral aspect of a left knee demonstrating the superficial layer of the iliotibial band and its iliopatellar band expansion.

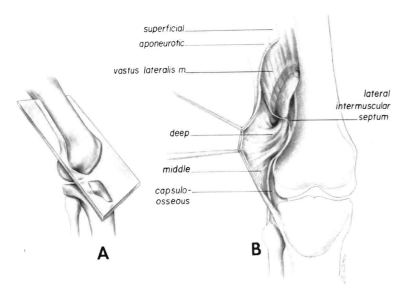

Figure 3–2   (A) Plane of section. **(B)** Coronal oblique illustration of the right knee demonstrating the course of the deep and capsulo-osseous layers of the iliotibial band. (From Terry GC, Hughston JC, Norwood LA. The anatomy of the iliopatellar band and iliotibial tract. Am J Sports Med 1986;14:39–45, with permission.)

The deep layer of the iliotibial band is medial to the superficial layer and attaches the medial aspect of the superficial layer to the distal aspect of the lateral intermuscular septum of the distal femur.[33,34] Deep and posterior to the deep and superficial layers of the iliotibial band, the capsulo-osseous layer of the iliotibial band emerges from deep and more proximal attachments to the lateral head of the gastrocnemius and short head of the biceps femoris muscle to attach just medial and distal to the deep layer of the iliotibial band along the supracondylar area of the lateral aspect of the femur[33,34] **(Fig. 3–2)**. From this proximal attachment site on the femur, as well as its attachment sites to these two muscle groups, the capsulo-osseous layer of the iliotibial band continues distally as a fascial sling over the lateral aspect of the joint. It attaches to the tibia just posterior and proximal to Gerdy's tubercle. This lateral-based sling is what one attempts to reconstruct in extraarticular anterior cruciate ligament reconstructions.

◆ Long Head of the Biceps Femoris

The long head of the biceps femoris forms the posterior aspect of the sheet of tissues that cover the lateral aspect of the knee. Overall, the long head of the biceps femoris has six attachments at the knee.[36–38] About a centimeter proximal to the lateral aspect of the fibular head and styloid, the long head of the biceps femoris tendon divides into two tendonous components. These are the direct arm and the anterior arm. The direct arm is the distal termination of the majority of the common biceps tendon and inserts on the far posterolateral edge of the fibular

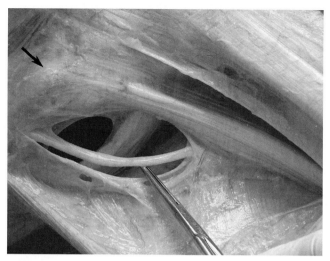

Figure 3–3 The lateral aspect of a left knee demonstrating the direct and anterior arms of the long head of the biceps femoris. Hemostat is pointing to the common peroneal nerve (arrow).

head, slightly lateral and distal to the tip of the fibular styloid **(Fig. 3–3)**. The anterior arm of the long biceps has a portion of its substance attaching slightly distolateral to the direct arm attachment on the posterolateral aspect of the fibular head, with the majority of the more lateral substance of the anterior arm continuing distally, where it crosses lateral to the fibular collateral ligament. In this location, a small bursa is located anterolateral to the distal fourth of the fibular collateral ligament. The anterior arm of the long head of the biceps femoris serves as the lateral wall of this bursa. It is a very useful clinical landmark because a small horizontal incision through the anterior arm, 1 cm proximal to the fibular head, allows for direct and consistent access to the attachment site of the fibular collateral ligament on the fibular head **(Fig. 3–4)**. This surgical approach is

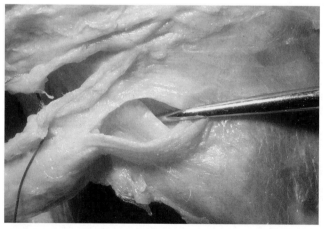

Figure 3–4 The lateral aspect of a right knee. The anterior arm of the long head of the biceps femoris has been incised to expose the fibular collateral ligament within the fibular collateral ligament/biceps femoris bursa.

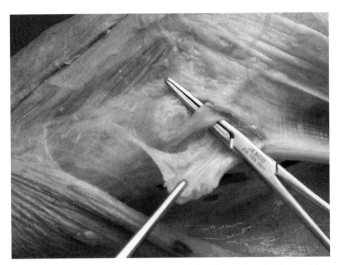

Figure 3–5 The components of the long head of the biceps femoris of a left knee (anterior arm is held in forceps, anterior aponeurosis continues down leg, lateral aponeurosis is deep to hemostat under [medial] fibular collatural ligament).

extremely useful in identifying the injured fibular collateral ligament during a repair or reconstruction. In addition, a suture placed into the substance of the fibular collateral ligament allows for traction to be placed on it and for easier identification of proximal tears, which may be encased in scar tissue or avulsed off the femur.[39]

In addition to these two tendonous components of the long head of the biceps femoris, there are four fascial components: a reflected arm, a lateral aponeurosis, an anterior aponeurosis, and a distal fascial expansion[36] **(Fig. 3–5)**.

After the anterior arm of the long head of the biceps crosses the fibular collateral ligament, it continues distally and anteriorly and terminates as an anterior aponeurosis over the anterior compartment of the leg. Proximal to the fibular attachment, the anterior edge of the anterior arm provides an attachment for a lateral aponeurotic expansion to the posterior and lateral aspect of the distal aspect of the fibular collateral ligament. In addition, a reflected arm of the long head of the biceps tendon ascends anteriorly, crosses the distal portion of the short head of the biceps femoris, just proximal to the direct arm fibular attachment, and attaches to the posterior edge of the superficial layer of the iliotibial tract. Finally, the posterior aspect of the long head of the biceps femoris tendon has a distal fascial expansion of tissues that attach to the lateral gastrocnemius and sulcus muscles.

The main components that are injured in posterolateral knee injuries are usually the two tendonous components, the direct arm, and the anterior arm. These structures may be avulsed off their fibular attachments and retracted proximally in severe posterolateral knee injuries. It is important to attempt to reconstitute their attachment on the lateral aspect of the fibular head to restore normal dynamic function to the biceps femoris complex. In addition, we attempt to repair the lateral aponeurosis back to the fibular collateral ligament in acute injuries so that the normal dynamic function that the biceps femoris has in relation to the fibular collateral ligament can be restored.

◆ Short Head of the Biceps Femoris Muscle

Although on gross observation it appears that the majority of the short head of the biceps femoris consists of the muscular attachment that courses down to attach to the common biceps tendon, it has several important attachments at the posterolateral corner of the knee. Overall, there are six attachments of the short head of the biceps femoris muscle at the knee.[36]

The short head of the biceps femoris muscle originates just medial to the linea aspera of the distal femur, and its muscle fibers extend anterior, distal, and lateral to attach to the medial edge of the common biceps tendon. The first attachment component of the short head of the biceps femoris at the knee is this proximal muscular attachment to the anterior and medial aspect of the common biceps tendon (**Fig. 3–6**).

A broad capsular attachment that extends from the short biceps tendon to several structures, including the posterolateral aspect of the lateral joint capsule, a bony or cartilaginous fabella or fabella analogue, and the lateral gastrocnemius complex, is called the capsular arm (**Fig. 3–7**). The capsular arm is the first main attachment that courses off the short head of the biceps femoris toward the posterolateral structures. This capsular arm is a main component of the biceps femoris complex, which attaches along the posterolateral aspect of the knee. It courses down along the short biceps tendon to attach to the tip of the fibular styloid and forms a large fascial sheath to attach to the posterolateral corner of the knee. In some former studies, the structure has been referred to as part of the "arcuate ligament."[15,18,19,23,24,26] The distal edge of the capsular arm of the short biceps is the fabellofibular ligament.[34]

Distal to the capsular arm of the short biceps, a third attachment of the short biceps at the knee forms a fascial confluence with the capsulo-osseous layer of the iliotibial band. This fascial confluence forms a Y-shaped anterolateral sling that courses medial to the superficial layer of the iliotibial band and the short head of the biceps femoris, and continues distally to attach on the

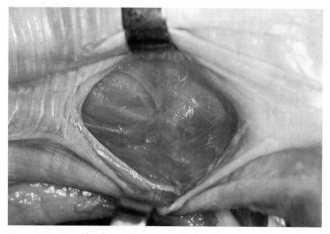

Figure 3–6 The lateral aspect of a right knee demonstrating the course of the main muscle fibers of the short head of the biceps femoris.

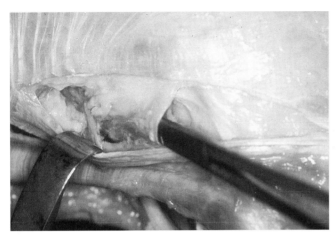

Figure 3–7 The lateral aspect of a right knee demonstrating the capsular arm of the short head of the biceps femoris (under hemostat) as it courses to the posterolateral capsule and lateral gastrocnemius complex (inferior aspect iliotibial band retracted).

proximolateral tibia just posterior to Gerdy's tubercle. This fascial sling has clinical significance in that it was the main component of the structures that were reconstructed in extraarticular anterior cruciate ligament reconstructions.

Once the short head of the biceps femoris reaches the fibular head and styloid region, there is a direct arm attachment that inserts just lateral to the tip of the fibular styloid (and medial to the direct arm attachment of the long head of the biceps femoris). A distinct tendinous attachment between the short and long heads of the biceps direct arm attachments on the lateral downslope of the fibular styloid can be well visualized on high-resolution magnetic resonance imaging (MRI) scans **(Fig. 3–8)**. In addition to the direct arm tendinous attachment, an anterior arm of the short head of the biceps femoris courses off just proximal to the fibular styloid attachment and passes medial to the fibular collateral ligament and inserts on the tibia 1 cm posterior to Gerdy's tubercle. This anterior arm attachment on the tibia is at the same location as the meniscotibial portion of the mid-third lateral capsular ligament (lateral capsule).[36] This attachment site can be well visualized on coronal high-resolution MRI scans, especially when there is an associated soft tissue avulsion or bony Segond fracture.[40]

The final attachment of the short head of the biceps femoris at the knee is the lateral aponeurotic expansion. This lateral aponeurotic expansion courses anterior and distal off the distal portion of the short head of the biceps femoris to attach to the posteromedial aspect of the fibular collateral ligament.

The main clinically relevant components of the short head of the biceps femoris at the knee are the capsular arm, the anterior arm, and the direct arm. The capsular arm has significance because of its broad fascial attachments over the posterolateral aspect of the knee. These components become lax in flexion and very tight in extension and have not been well studied biomechanically. One of the most common sites of injury that we see is that of components avulsed off the fibular attachment, and we attempt to repair them when they are avulsed in this location. Most commonly, they are avulsed with a tear of the

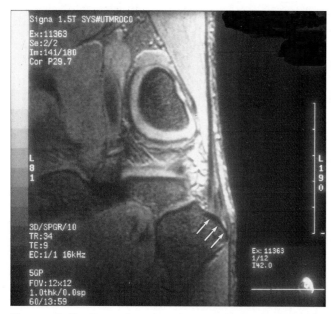

Figure 3–8 Coronal magnetic resonance imaging (MRI) scan of a left knee demonstrating the distinct attachment sites of the direct arms of the short and long heads of the biceps femoris and the anterior arm of the long head (arrows).

direct arm of the short biceps femoris off the fibular head, with or without a concurrent avulsion of the attachment sites of the direct and anterior arms of the long head of the biceps femoris.[41] In these instances, we attempt to repair them back to their anatomic attachment sites on the lateral downslope of the fibular styloid. The most common location that we see with an anterior arm injury is that of an avulsion off the tibia concurrent with a bony or soft tissue Segond injury. In these instances, we attempt a direct repair back to the tibia when we are doing a surgical approach for an acute injury. Because these structures are tight in extension, it would appear that they are functionally important to the prevention of knee hyperextension.

◆ Fibular Collateral Ligament

The fibular, or lateral, collateral ligament is one of the three main structures that provide static stability to the lateral and posterolateral aspect of the knee. It has an important role both in providing varus stability at all knee flexion angles and in providing external rotation stability in the early phases of knee flexion. It is the main primary static stabilizer to varus opening in the knee (see Chapter 6). All biomechanical tests to date have shown no statistically significant increase in varus opening of the knee, even when all of the posterolateral structures and the cruciate ligaments are cut, until the fibular collateral ligament has also been sectioned.[22–44]

In this regard, I believe it is very important to attempt either an anatomic primary repair or a reconstruction of this important stabilizer of the posterolateral corner of the knee. We have performed both qualitative and quantitative studies of the attachment sites of the fibular collateral ligament to help in understanding its anatomic position.[32,34]

Qualitatively, the fibular collateral ligament originates from the femur with a fan-like attachment site that is slightly proximal and posterior to the lateral epicondyle. It is extremely important to recognize that the fibular collateral ligament does not have a direct attachment to the lateral epicondyle.[32,36] It has an average femoral attachment site that is slightly proximal (1.4 mm) and posterior (3.1 mm) to the lateral epicondyle[32] **(Fig. 3–9)**.

After its attachment site on the femur, the fibular collateral ligament then courses over the lateral aspect of the knee to attach to the lateral aspect of the fibular head. Along its course, it passes medial to the superficial layer of the iliotibial band and the reflected arm of the long head of the biceps femoris. In

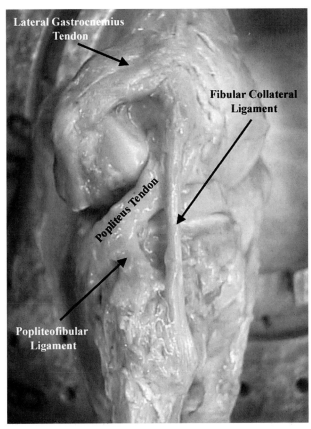

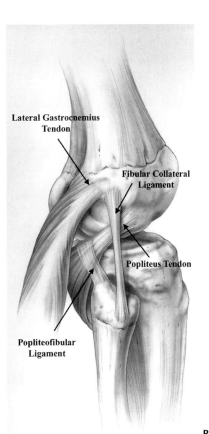

Figure 3–9 Photograph **(A)** and drawing **(B)** of the lateral aspect of a right knee demonstrating the course and attachment sites of the fibular collateral ligament. (From LaPrade RF, Ly TV, Wentorf FA, Engebretsen L. The posterolateral attachments of the knee: a qualitative and quantitative morphologic analysis of the fibular collateral ligament, popliteus tendon, popliteofibular ligament, and lateral gastrocnemius tendon. Am J Sports Med 2003;31: 854–860, with permission.)

addition, the lateral aponeurotic expansions of the short and long heads of the biceps femoris attach along its posterior border in its distal course. The distal quarter of the fibular collateral ligament is exposed along its lateral and anterior aspects within the fibular collateral ligament–biceps bursa.[37] The anterior arm of the long head of the biceps femoris crosses the lateral aspect of the fibular collateral ligament along this portion of its distal course. As noted previously, this is an important site to identify the fibular collateral ligament intraoperatively for both surgical repairs and reconstructions.

After it passes through the biceps bursa, the fibular collateral ligament has its main fibers attached to the lateral aspect of the fibular head. Some of the more lateral fibers of the fibular collateral ligament are continuous with the superficial fascia of the peroneus longus muscle of the leg and have the appearance of continuing distal to this. This does have some clinical significance in that there are times when the fibular collateral ligament can be peeled off the lateral aspect of the fibula and can demonstrate instability on clinical examination but does not appear to be disrupted on coronal MRI scans because of its continuous attachment with this lateral compartment fascia. This is important to identify at the time of surgical repair; to do so, identify the fibular collateral ligament attachment on the fibular head through the biceps bursa and tug on it to assess for any distal attachment site injury.

The fibular collateral ligament is noted to attach slightly anterior to the midportion of the lateral aspect of the fibular head. Overall, it attaches at an average of 38% of the width of the fibular head from anterior to posterior along its lateral aspect. In addition, it attaches at an average of 8.2 mm posterior to the anterior aspect of the fibular head and 28.4 mm distal to the tip of the fibular styloid.[32]

Clinically, the anatomic attachment sites help to identify why attempted isometric reconstructions of the fibular collateral ligament in the past have not worked. These "isometric" attempts at reconstruction did not place the reconstruction grafts into their anatomic positions, which helps to explain the differences in graft excursion at these sites.

◆ Mid-Third Lateral Capsular Ligament

The mid-third lateral capsular ligament is the thickening of the lateral capsule of the knee joint and is equivalent to the deep medial collateral ligament on the medial aspect of the knee.[34,39] It is basically the capsule that attaches on the femur and courses down to the tibia over the lateral aspect of the knee. Its anterior attachment on the femur is formed along a line from anterior and proximal to the lateral epicondyle to its posterior edge at the supracondylar process of the lateral femoral condyle. Along this thin line of capsular attachment, it attaches to the posterior aspect of the popliteus attachment on the femur and courses back posterior to end at the lateral gastrocnemius tendon attachment on the femur (**Fig. 3–10**). It also is intimately involved with the fibular collateral ligament and its femoral attachment site.

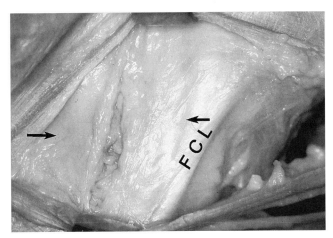

Figure 3–10 the mid-third lateral capsular ligament of the left knee (incised, arrows). The superficial layer of iliotibial band is retracted; the fibular collateral ligament (FCL) is seen posteriorly.

The mid-third lateral capsular ligament courses distally from its femoral attachment site to attach on the tibia just distal to the lateral tibial plateau articular cartilage margin. It attaches anteriorly just posterior to Gerdy's tubercle and its posterior boundary is at the anterior edge of the popliteal hiatus.

The mid-third lateral capsular ligament has two distinct components. The meniscofemoral ligament comprises the portion that courses between its femoral attachment and the superior aspect of the lateral meniscus at this location, whereas the meniscotibial ligament is that portion that courses from the inferior border of the lateral meniscus to its tibial attachment site.[34,40]

◆ Fabellofibular Ligament

The fabellofibular ligament is one of the most misunderstood structures over the posterolateral aspect of the knee. Part of the reason for it being misunderstood is the difficulty in isolating it in cadaveric formalin-preserved knees. In addition, the structure is tight in knee extension, but most knees are dissected with the knee in flexion where the structure appears to be less substantial. It is important to understand exactly what this structure does in its course to understand how to isolate it and what its purpose may be.

By definition, the fabellofibular ligament is the distal edge of the capsular arm of the short head of the biceps femoris, and as such it is present in all knees.[34,39] However, it is noted in knees with a bony fabella that this structure is more substantial than in those knees with either a cartilaginous fabella analogue or just a thin substance of thickened capsule in this area.[4,14,15]

The fabellofibular ligament originates along the lateral aspect of the fabella, or a cartilaginous fabella analogue, and descends distally and laterally to attach just lateral to the tip of the fibular styloid. It is most readily identified on high-

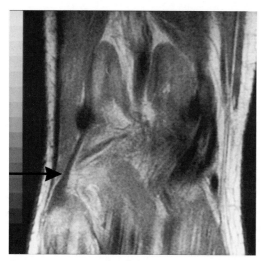

Figure 3–11 Coronal MRI scan of a right knee demonstrating the fabellofibular ligament as it courses from the tip of the fibular styloid to the fabella and lateral capsule at this location.

resolution MRI scans on the coronal imaging sequences at the far posterior tip of the fibular styloid[40] (**Fig. 3–11**).

As part of our attempt to understand this structure, we performed dissections on the fabellas present in 100 knees. To do this, we dissected out the posterolateral capsule in formalin-preserved cadavers, isolated out the fabella region, obtained radiographs of all the fabellas, and performed histologic staining for proteoglycans in all of them. We found a distinct bony fabella in 38% of knees. In the remaining 62% there was a variable amount of proteoglycan staining, which identified them all as having a cartilaginous fabella. In some instances, there was a definite palpable fabella, which did not have any different features to distinguish it from a bony fabella except by radiographs. It was noted that in all instances a fabella could be isolated from the lateral capsule. In those knees in which there was no substantial fabella noted on palpation, I found that by inverting the posterolateral capsule there was always a portion of this posterolateral capsule, between 8 and 10 mm in size, that maintained a concave surface where the lateral gastrocnemius tendon attached along with the plantaris muscle. Histologic staining through this area always revealed positive staining for proteoglycan on Safranin-O stains. Thus I feel comfortable in stating that a cartilaginous fabella appears to be present in all knees, even in those where there is no bony fabella.

The clinical significance of the fabellofibular ligament is that it appears to be important for providing stability of the knee close to extension. Although biomechanical studies have not been performed to date to help identify which posterior structures are important in preventing hyperextension of the knee when the cruciate ligaments and medial collateral and fibular collateral ligaments are intact, one can infer that this structure may have some significance. Thus when treating an acute operative posterolateral knee injury, we attempt to restore the integrity of the direct arm of the short head of the biceps femoris and the capsular arm of the short head of the biceps femoris/fabellofibular ligament complex attachment on the tip of the fibular styloid to restore their combined static and dynamic function to the posterolateral corner of the knee.

◆ Coronary Ligament of the Lateral Meniscus

The coronary ligament of the lateral meniscus is the meniscotibial portion of the posterior joint capsule that attaches the posterior horn of the lateral meniscus to the tibia.[17,23,34] Its lateral border is at the edge of the posteroinferior popliteomeniscal fascicle at the popliteal hiatus, and the more medial border is just lateral to the posterior cruciate ligament attachment on the posterior cruciate ligament facet of the tibia. The coronary ligament is reinforced along its entire length by the aponeurotic attachment of the popliteus muscle to the lateral meniscus[34] **(Fig. 3–12)**.

This structure is thought to be important clinically to provide resistance to hyperextension and posterolateral rotation of the knee. It seems to be more important due to the combined effect of the popliteal aponeurosis and its attachment to the coronary ligament and posterolateral capsule. In the past, this was noted to be an important part of the arcuate ligament[16] as well as in providing some important function to preventing a positive reverse pivot shift test.[45] It can be very difficult to approach this structure surgically, and I prefer to identify lesions on it by first performing an arthroscopy of the lateral compartment of the knee to determine if

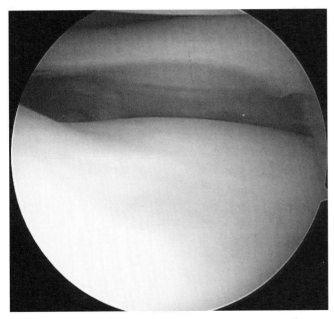

Figure 3–12 Arthroscopic view demonstrating the coronary ligament of the posterior horn of the lateral meniscus (left knee, patient with lateral compartment drive-through sign).

dissection in the interval between the lateral gastrocnemius and soleus over to this portion of the knee is necessary in those patients with acute knee injuries.

◆ Popliteus Muscle Complex at the Knee

In addition to the fibular collateral ligament, the components of the popliteus muscle complex comprise the most important structures for static stability in the posterolateral knee.[43,44,46,47] The popliteus muscle complex is a very complex series of interactions among its eight components at the knee. This complex consists of the popliteus tendon attachment on the femur, the three popliteomeniscal fascicles (anteroinferior, posterosuperior, and posteroinferior), the popliteofibular ligament (with its anterior and posterior divisions), the aponeurotic attachment to the posterior capsule and posterior horn of the lateral meniscus, and the popliteus muscle belly itself.[32,34,39]

The popliteus tendon femoral attachment has a constant broad-based attachment at the most proximal and anterior fifth of the popliteal sulcus. In this location, the popliteus tendon's femoral attachment is always anterior to the fibular collateral ligament's femoral attachment (**Fig. 3–13**). Our quantitative studies have also demonstrated that the average distance between the midpoints of the femoral attachment sites of the popliteus tendon and fibular collateral ligament is 18.5 mm[32] (**Fig. 3–14**). This rather large distance is important to recognize when one is attempting either a primary repair or a reconstructive procedure of these two structures. One can see that because of the differences in their attachment locations, and the large distances between them, one repair site or reconstructive bone plug would create more of a sling procedure than an actual reconstruction for these two structures.[48]

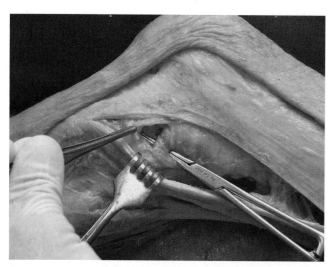

Figure 3–13   The lateral aspect of a right knee demonstrating the location of the popliteus tendon attachment (under hemostat) on the femur.

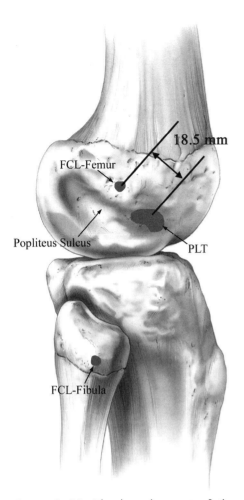

Figure 3–14 The lateral aspect of the right knee demonstrating the 18.5-mm distance between the popliteus tendon (PLT) and the fibular collateral ligament femoral attachment sites. (From LaPrade RF, Ly TV, Wentorf FA, Engebretsen L. The posterolateral attachments of the knee: a qualitative and quantitative morphologic analysis of the fibular collateral ligament, popliteus tendon, popliteofibular ligament, and lateral gastrocnemius tendon. Am J Sports Med 2003;31:854–860, with permission.)

After the popliteus tendon attaches on the femur, it is noted to course intraarticularly and distally into the popliteal hiatus. It should be noted that the popliteus tendon does not fully engage into the full confines of the popliteal sulcus until the knee is flexed to 112 degrees.[32] In addition, there is a small sinusoidal indentation of the articular cartilage of the lateral femoral condyle that is made by the popliteus tendon when the knee is in full extension. Stäubli and Birrer[23] called this the sulcus statorius of Fürst. The significance of why the popliteus tendon does not fully engage into the popliteal sulcus until 112 degrees of knee flexion is unknown.

As the popliteus tendon courses into the popliteal hiatus, it attaches to the lateral meniscus via the anteroinferior, posterosuperior, and posteroinferior

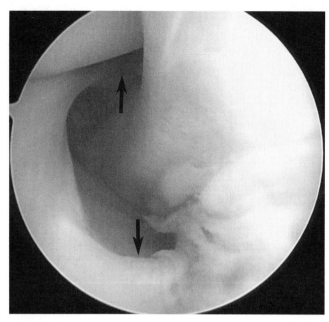

Figure 3–15 Arthroscopic view, left knee, demonstrating the "hoop-like" attachment of the anteroinferior popliteomeniscal fascicle (foreground) (top arrow) and the posterosuperior popliteomeniscal fascicle (bottom arrow) to the lateral meniscus.

popliteomeniscal fascicles.[23,24,34] These meniscal fascicles form a "hoop-like" attachment from the popliteus tendon to the lateral meniscus at the popliteal hiatus **(Fig. 3–15)**. These fascicles are thought to be important in providing stability to the lateral meniscus and preventing medial entrapment of the lateral meniscus with functional varus forces to the knee.[49] It is thought that the anteroinferior popliteomeniscal fascicle is the most important attachment of the popliteus complex to the lateral meniscus.[49]

Further down the popliteus tendon, the popliteofibular ligament originates at the popliteus musculotendinous junction, just distal to the popliteomeniscal fascicles.[23,32] The popliteofibular ligament courses slightly distally and laterally to attach to the medial aspect of the fibular styloid. The popliteofibular ligament has two divisions[23,32,34] **(Fig. 3–16)**. The anterior division attaches on the anteromedial downslope of the fibular styloid. In this location, it also blends with the distal edge of the anteroinferior popliteomeniscal fascicle and also with the fibers connecting the anteroproximal tibiofibular joint. There are also attachments to the tibia in this location because of its proximity to the proximal tibiofibular joint. The posterior division of the popliteofibular ligament attaches to the posteromedial downslope of the fibular styloid.

The posterior division of the popliteofibular ligament appears to have more substance and is thought to provide a more important function to static stability of the posterolateral corner of the knee than the anterior division. The

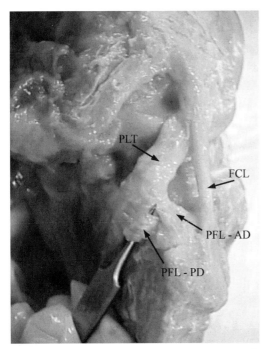

Figure 3–16 The posterolateral aspect of the right knee demonstrating the posterior and anterior divisions (PD, AD) of the popliteofibular ligament (PFL). (From LaPrade RF, Ly TV, Wentorf FA, Engebretsen L. The posterolateral attachments of the knee: a qualitative and quantitative morphologic analysis of the fibular collateral ligament, popliteus tendon, popliteofibular ligament, and lateral gastrocnemius tendon. Am J Sports Med 2003;31:854–860, with permission.)

average width of the posterior division's attachment on the fibular styloid is 5.8 mm, whereas the average width of the anterior division's attachment on the fibular styloid is 2.6 mm.[32]

Coursing distally past the musculotendinous junction of the popliteus complex, a broad aponeurotic attachment extends from the popliteus muscle belly to the posterolateral joint capsule, coronary ligament, and the posterior horn of the lateral meniscus.[16,34] As noted in the section on the coronary ligament, this portion of the popliteus complex has been called the arcuate ligament in the past,[16] and has also been noted to provide some importance in preventing a positive reverse pivot shift test.[45]

Deep to the popliteal aponeurosis to the lateral meniscus, there is a thickening of the posterior joint capsule, which I have called the proximal popliteal capsular expansion. It connects the posteromedial knee capsule at its intercondylar notch attachment to the medial aspect of the popliteus musculotendinous junction (**Fig. 3–17**). The proximal posterior popliteus capsular expansion averages 40.5 mm long and courses anterior to the oblique popliteal ligament. Its functional significance is not known, but it is noted to become quite stout with rotation of the knee. In addition, there is noted to be a direct attachment from the posteromedial aspect of the joint to the fibular head and styloid,

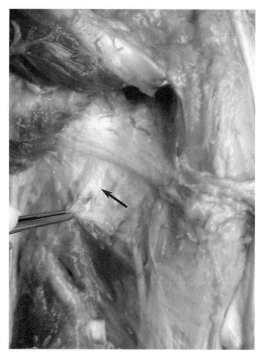

Figure 3–17 The posterior view of a left knee. The proximal popliteal capsular expansion (arrow) is noted in the pickups.

through the popliteofibular ligament, and through this attachment to the posteromedial joint capsule.

Distal to the popliteal aponeurosis to the lateral meniscus and the proximal popliteal capsular expansion are the main fibers of the popliteus muscle, which continues its distomedial course and attaches to the posteromedial edge of the middle to distal posterior tibia. In this location, the popliteus muscle belly is covered posteriorly by the distal tibial expansion of the semimembranosus complex. This distal tibial expansion is located just posterior to the tibial collateral ligament, and has two divisions, one medial and the other lateral, with a connecting fascial layer coursing between each division that forms a fascial expansion over the popliteus muscle.

◆ Lateral Gastrocnemius Tendon

The lateral gastrocnemius tendon forms at the far lateral edge of the lateral gastrocnemius muscle belly. Along its course, it attaches to a fabella, or a cartilaginous fabella analogue, which has been found to be present in all knees.[34] Proximal to the fabella region, the lateral gastrocnemius tendon attaches to and is inseparable from the meniscofemoral portion of the posterior capsule

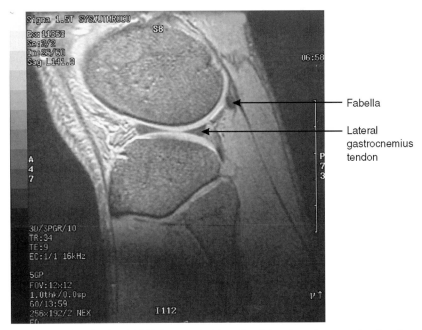

Fabella

Lateral
gastrocnemius
tendon

Figure 3–18 Sagittal MRI demonstrating the lateral gastrocnemius tendon and its relationship to the fabella and the meniscofemoral portion of the posterior capsule (left knee).

(Fig. 3–18). We have performed histologic studies in this area and note that the fibers of the lateral gastrocnemius tendon and the meniscofemoral portion of the posterior capsule proximal to the fabella region are inseparable. Thus one can see why it is difficult to dissect along this layer for a lateral meniscus repair or other approach to this portion of the knee. In effect, it is impossible to split the lateral gastrocnemius tendon away from the posterior capsule proximal to the fabella, and when one does so there is a high likelihood of either entering the joint or separating the tendon away from the main fibers of its muscle belly.

The lateral gastrocnemius tendon femoral attachment is in the region of the supracondylar process. In our anatomy studies, it is consistently noted to attach near or at the supracondylar process of the distal femur. Its average attachment site is 13.8 mm posterior to the fibular collateral ligament's femoral attachment site.[32]

The clinical importance of the lateral gastrocnemius tendon lies in the fact that we have found it to be rarely injured in posterolateral knee injuries.[47] In addition, the lateral gastrocnemius tendon has been included in bony advancement or recess procedures of a posterolateral knee bone block with its associated femoral attachment sites of the lateral gastrocnemius tendon, fibular collateral ligament, and popliteus tendon.[50–52] In addition, it also serves as a useful reference point to help identify the normal attachment site of the fibular collateral ligament when there is an acute or chronic avulsion of its attachment site on the femur.

◆ Inferior Lateral Genicular Artery

The inferior lateral genicular artery is an important landmark structure for the posterolateral corner of the knee. We have found that identifying it on MRI scans assists in differentiating between the attachment sites of the fabellofibular and popliteofibular ligament on the fibular head and styloid.[40] Clinically it is important to identify this artery along its course during a surgical approach or repair so that it can be properly coagulated (if necessary), preventing a significant postoperative hematoma.

The inferior lateral genicular artery originates off the popliteal artery and courses along the posterior joint capsule just proximal to the superior aspect of the lateral meniscus. From this location, it courses laterally to pass posterior to the popliteofibular ligament and anterior to the fabellofibular ligament attachment sites on the fibula.[4,14,19,23,24,34] From this location, it then courses anterior to pass directly along the lateral aspect of the meniscus within the substance of the mid-third lateral capsular ligament. It is important to recognize this meniscus when making a lateral capsular arthrotomy incision in that the artery will be present right at the level of the meniscus and should be identified and coagulated in all instances to minimize postoperative bleeding.

◆ Oblique Popliteal Ligament

The oblique popliteal ligament courses over both the posteromedial and the posterolateral aspect of the knee. It forms a broad fascial sheath over the posterior aspect of the knee with an average length of 48.0 mm and an average width medially of 9.5 mm and laterally of 16.4 mm. It is noted to be formed medially by a coalescence of the capsular arm of the posterior oblique ligament and a lateral tendinous expansion off the common semimembranosus tendon. Laterally, the oblique popliteal ligament attaches on the meniscofemoral portion of the lateral capsule, confluent with the plantaris muscle attachment on the lateral aspect of a bony or cartilaginous fabella **(Fig. 3–19)**. We have found this attachment site to be contrary to some anatomy textbooks and published literature that have reported that the oblique popliteal ligament's lateral attachment site is on the posterior aspect of the femur.[16,18,53,54] In fact, the proximal edge of the oblique popliteal ligament's lateral attachment averages 19.0 mm distal to the posterior capsule's femoral attachment at this site. Therefore, in this location, the oblique popliteal ligament has a common attachment site with the fabellofibular ligament and the capsular arm of the short head of the biceps, as well as with the lateral gastrocnemius tendon complex that attaches to the fabella. This attachment relationship does help to explain why the oblique popliteal ligament (medially) and the fabellofibular ligament, capsular arm of the short head of the biceps femoris, and the popliteofibular ligament (laterally) were often lumped together and called the arcuate ligament in earlier studies because together they formed an arched-like appearance over the posterior aspect of the knee.

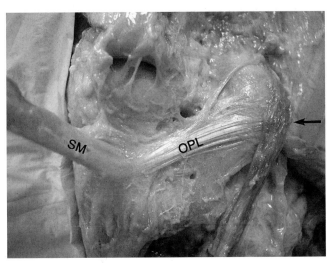

Figure 3–19   The posterior view of a right knee demonstrating the oblique popliteal ligament (OPL). Medially, it is formed by a coalescence of the capsular arm of the posterior oblique ligament and a lateral tendonous expansion off the common semimembranosus tendon (SM). Laterally, it attaches to the lateral capsule in the region of the fabella and the plantaris muscle attachment (arrow) (medial and lateral heads of gastrocnemius removed, plantaris muscle in situ).

◆ The Arcuate Ligament

The arcuate ligament is not a single, distinct ligament, but actually is several structures that combine to form an arched, or "arcuate," appearance when viewed qualitatively from posterior over the posterolateral aspect of the knee. To prevent confusion, I have recommended that the term *arcuate ligament* not be utilized in the future and that we rely solely on the individual anatomic structures. For those of us who are splitters rather than lumpers, this would be similar to using the term *patellofemoral pain* in patients who may have either patellar tendonopathy, patellofemoral chondromalacia, medial plical irritation, or pes anserine bursitis.

In any event, there do appear to be two limbs due to the qualitative appearance of an arched ligament. The medial limb of the arched ligament is formed by the oblique popliteal ligament.[34] The oblique popliteal ligament is formed over the medial side of the knee by a coalescence of the oblique popliteal expansion of the semimembranosus muscle and the capsular arm of the posterior oblique ligament and then these structures course over the posterolateral aspect of the knee to attach along the posterolateral capsule and at the lateral aspect of the fabella. The lateral limb of the arched ligament is composed of those structures that course from the posteromedial aspect of the fibular styloid to attach to the posterolateral capsule. These structures consist of the popliteofibular ligament, fabellofibular ligament, and the capsular arm of the short head of the biceps femoris.[34,39]

As I have noted previously, there is significant confusion about which structure comprises the arcuate ligament and significant variation in the literature among multiple different sources. It is strongly recommended that the term "arcuate ligament" not be utilized in the future to verify that anatomists and clinicians refer to the same structures in their descriptions of the posterolateral knee.

References

1. Fürst CM. Der Musculus Popliteus und Seine Sehne. Ueber ihre Entwicklung und uber Einige Damit Zusammenhangende Bildungen. Lunds Universitets Arsskrift Band 39, Lund, Germany: E. Malstroms Buchdruckerei, 1903 (German)
2. Herzmark MH. The evolution of the knee joint. J Bone Joint Surg 1938;20:77–84
3. Haines RW. The tetrapod knee joint. J Anat 1942;76:270–301
4. Kaplan EB. The fabellofibular and short lateral ligaments of the knee joint. J Bone Joint Surg 1961;43A:169–179
5. Taylor G, Bonney V. On the homology and morphology of the popliteus muscle: a contribution to comparative myology. J Anat Physiol 1905;40:34–50
6. Fabbriciani C, Oransky M, Zoppi U. The popliteal muscle: an anatomical study. Arch Ital Anat Embriol 1982;87:203–217
7. Kaplan EB. The iliotibial tract: clinical and morphological significance. J Bone Joint Surg 1958;40A:817–832
8. Kaplan EB. Comparative anatomy of the extensor digitorum longus in relation to the knee joint. Anat Rec 1958B;131:129–149
9. Marshall JL, Girgis FG, Zelko RR. The biceps femoris tendon and its functional significance. J Bone Joint Surg 1972;54A:1444–1450
10. Crum JA, LaPrade RF, Wentorf FA. The anatomy of the posterolateral aspect of the rabbit knee. J Orthop Res 2003;21:723–729
11. Maissiat JH. Etudes de Physique Animale. Paris: Bethune et Plon, 1843 (French)
12. Dujarier C. Anatomie des Membres; Dissection; Anatomie Topographique, Paris: G. Steinheil, 1905 (French)
13. Vallois HV. Etudes Anatomiques de L'articulation du Genou Ches les Primates. Thesis, Universite de Montpellier, No. 63, 1914 (French)
14. Seebacher JR, Inglis AE, Marshall JL, Warren RF. The structure of the posterolateral aspect of the knee. J Bone Joint Surg 1982;64A:536–541
15. Sudasna S, Harnsiriwattanagit K. The ligamentous structures of the posterolateral aspect of the knee. Bull Hosp Joint Dis 1990;50:35–40
16. Last RJ. Some anatomical details of the knee joint. J Bone Joint Surg 1948;30B:683–688
17. Last RJ. The popliteus muscle and the lateral meniscus: with a note on the attachment of the medial meniscus. J Bone Joint Surg 1950;32B:93–99
18. Kaplan EB. Surgical approach to the lateral (peroneal) side of the knee joint. Surg Gynel Obstet 1957;104:346–356
19. Watanabe Y, Moriya H, Takahashi K, et al. Functional anatomy of the posterolateral structures of the knee. Arthroscopy 1993;9:57–62
20. Lovejoy JF, Harden TT. Popliteus muscle in man. Anat Rec 1971;169:727–730
21. Hughston JC, Andrews JR, Cross MJ, Moschi A. Classification of knee ligament instabilities. Part II: the lateral compartment. J Bone Joint Surg 1976;58A:173–179

22. Müller W. The Knee: Form, Function and Ligament Reconstruction. New York: Springer-Verlag, 1983

23. Stäubli HU, Birrer S. The popliteus tendon and its fascicles at the popliteus hiatus: gross anatomy and functional arthroscopic evaluation with and without anterior cruciate ligament deficiency. Arthroscopy 1990;6:209–220

24. Stäubli HU, Rauschning W. Popliteus tendon and lateral meniscus: gross and multiplanar cryosectional anatomy of the knee. Am J Knee Surg 1991;4:110–121

25. Hughston KC. Knee Ligaments. Injury and Repairs. Chicago: Mosby, 1993

26. Maynard MJ, Deng X-H, Wickiewicz TL, Warren RF. The popliteofibular ligament: rediscovery of a key element in posterolateral instability. Am J Sports Med 1996;24:311–316

27. Sutton JB. On the nature of certain ligaments. J Anat Physiol 1884;18:225–238

28. Higgins H. The popliteus muscle. J Anat 1894;29:569–573

29. Kaplan EB. Some aspects of functional anatomy of the human knee joint. Clin Orthop Rel Res 1962;23:18–29

30. Reis FP, Ferraz de Carvalho CA. Anatomical study on the proximal attachments of the human popliteus muscle. Rev Bras de Pesq Med e Biol 1975;8:373–380

31. Cohn AK, Mains DB. Popliteal hiatus of the lateral meniscus. Am J Sports Med 1979;7:221–226

32. LaPrade RF, Ly TV, Wentorf FA, Engebretsen L. The posterolateral attachments of the knee: a qualitative and quantitative morphologic analysis of the fibular collateral ligament, popliteus tendon, popliteofibular ligament, and lateral gastrocnemius tendon. Am J Sports Med 2003;31:854–860

33. Terry GC, Hughston JC, Norwood LA. The anatomy of the iliopatellar band and iliotibial tract. Am J Sports Med 1986;14:39–45

34. Terry GC, LaPrade RF. The posterolateral aspect of the knee: anatomy and surgical approach. Am J Sports Med 1996;24:732–739

35. Hughston JC, Flandry F, Brinker MR, Terry GC, Mills JC III. Surgical correction of medial subluxation of the patella. Am J Sports Med 1996;24:486–491

36. Terry GC, LaPrade RF. The biceps femoris muscle complex at the knee: its anatomy and injury patterns associated with acute anterolateral-anteromedial rotatory instability. Am J Sports Med 1996;24:2–8

37. LaPrade RF, Hamilton CD. The fibular collateral ligament–biceps femoris bursa: an anatomic study. Am J Sports Med 1997;25:439–443

38. LaPrade RF, Hamilton CD, Engebretsen L. Treatment of acute and chronic combined anterior cruciate ligament and posterolateral knee ligament injuries. Sports Med Arth Rev 1997;5:91–99

39. LaPrade RF. The medial collateral ligament complex and posterolateral aspect of the knee. In: Sports Medicine Orthopaedic Knowledge Update (OKU). Chicago: American Academy of Orthopaedic Surgeons, 1999

40. LaPrade RF, Gilbert TJ, Bollom TS, Wentorf FA, Chaljub G. The magnetic resonance imaging appearance of individual structures of the posterolateral knee: a prospective study of normal knees and knees with surgically verified grade III injuries. Am J Sports Med 2000;28:191–199

41. LaPrade RF, Terry GC. Injuries to the posterolateral aspect of the knee: association of anatomic injury patterns with clinical instability. Am J Sports Med 1997;25:433–438

42. Nielsen S, Ovesen J, Rasmussen O. The posterior cruciate ligament and rotatory knee stability: an experimental study. Arch Orthop Trauma Surg 1985;104:53–56

43. Gollehon DL, Torzilli PA, Warren RF. The role of the posterolateral and cruciate ligaments in the stability of the human knee: a biomechanical study. J Bone Joint Surg 1987;69A:233–242

44. Grood ES, Stowers SF, Noyes FR. Limits of movement in the human knee: effect of sectioning the posterior cruciate ligament and posterolateral structures. J Bone Joint Surg 1988;70A:88–97

45. Jakob RP, Hassler H, Stäubli HU. Observations on rotatory instability of the lateral compartment of the knee: experimental studies on the functional anatomy and pathomechanism of the true and reversed pivot shift sign. Acta Orthop Scand Suppl 1981;191:1–32

46. Nielsen S, Helmig P. The static stabilizing function of the popliteal tendon in the knee: an experimental study. Arch Orthop Trauma Surg 1986B;104:357–362

47. Veltri DM, Deng X-H, Torzilli PA, Warren RF, Maynard MJ. The role of the cruciate and posterolateral ligaments in stability of the knee. Am J Sports Med 1995;23:436–443

48. LaPrade RF, Johansen S, Wentorf FA, Engebretsen L, Esterberg JL, Tso A. An analysis of an anatomic posterolateral knee reconstruction: an *in vitro* biomechanical study and development of a surgical technique. Am J Sports Med 2004;32:1405–1414

49. Simonian PT, Sussman PS, van Trommel M, Wickiewicz TL, Warren RF. Popliteomeniscal fasciculi and lateral meniscal stability. Am J Sports Med 1997;25:849–853

50. Fleming RE, Blatz DJ, McCarroll JR. Posterior problems in the knee: posterior cruciate insufficiency and posterolateral rotatory insufficiency. Am J Sports Med 1981;9:107–113

51. Hughston JC, Jacobson KE. Chronic posterolateral rotatory instability of the knee. J Bone Joint Surg 1985;67A:351–359

52. Noyes FR, Barber-Westin SD. Surgical restoration to treat chronic deficiency of the posterolateral complex and cruciate ligaments of the knee joint. Am J Sports Med 1996;24:415–426

53. Winslow JB. An Anatomical Exposition of the Structure of the Human Body. London, 1733

54. Soames RW. Skeletal system. In: Gray's Anatomy. New York: Churchill Livingstone, 1995:703

4

Mechanism and Presenting History of Posterolateral Knee Injuries

The usual mechanism of injury of the posterolateral corner involves a component of contact or noncontact twisting, hyperextension, or varus force due to athletic injuries, falls, or motor vehicle accidents.[1-4] Historically, the main mechanism of injury has been reported to be a blow to the anteromedial aspect of the knee while the foot is firmly planted on the ground,[1,3] which results in a varus or varus/hyperextension knee injury (**Fig. 4–1**).

Although isolated posterolateral knee injuries would primarily occur due to a varus or posterolateral twisting mechanism, as it is at this position that increased stress is seen on the main static stabilizers of the knee,[5-8] it is recognized that most posterolateral knee injuries occur in combination with other ligament injuries, as these mechanisms of injury often cause injury to other knee ligaments and not just the posterolateral knee structures. Müller[9] noted that the popliteus tendon and the posterior cruciate ligament were parallel to each other, and that a tear of the posterior cruciate ligament was commonly associated with the posterolateral corner injury. The largest study population that recorded the mechanism of injury for posterolateral knee injuries (71 patients), reported that the most common mechanisms of injury were twisting (30%), noncontact hyperextension (21%), contact hyperextension (15%), an anterior blow to a flexed knee (10%), and a valgus force to a flexed knee (7%).[4] In this study, only 28% of these injuries were isolated grade 3 posterolateral corner knee injuries, with the remainder occurring in combination with other knee ligament injuries.[4]

It is important to recognize that many different mechanisms cause injuries to the structures of the posterolateral corner of the knee. Therefore, in addition to understanding the history of the etiology of these knee ligament injuries, it is also essential to verify the integrity of the posterolateral knee via a thorough clinical examination.

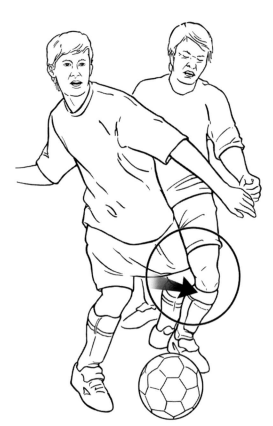

Figure 4–1 A classic mechanism of posterolateral knee injuries is a blow to the anteromedial aspect with the foot planted.

A thorough history must be obtained in patients with posterolateral knee injuries. Patients with acute isolated, or combined, ligament injuries may complain of pain along the posterolateral aspect of the knee.[4,10,11] Often, there is minimal swelling present, even in the face of an acute injury.[4] In addition to a thorough history that attempts to ascertain the mechanism of injury and any subjective patient complaints of instability, a thorough examination of the patellofemoral and tibiofemoral joint for knee instability, compared with the normal contralateral knee, must be performed.

Patients may also complain of numbness, dysesthesias, or distal motor weakness (including a footdrop) due to a neuropraxia or complete injury to the common peroneal nerve. It is especially important to determine the presence of these symptoms, even if transitory, as they may indicate that a significant varus or combined varus-rotational injury occurred to the knee. In addition, it is important to thoroughly document the neuromotor function of the common peroneal nerve prior to any surgical intervention so that postoperative circulation can be motor, and sensory follow-up exams are not confusing. Less than 50% of patients with a complete motor loss regain function over time, and it is important to discuss this frankly with patients at their initial presentation.

Patients with posterolateral knee injuries frequently describe instability with normal level walking, turning while climbing flights of stairs, or twisting, pivoting, or cutting to the affected side of the knee. Although the more severe varus-thrust gait pattern is more commonly seen with combined concurrent cruciate ligament injuries, it also can be seen in some athletes with an isolated acute, or chronic, fibular collateral ligament tear and a constitutional varus alignment. I examined a high school varsity quarterback with an isolated fibular collateral ligament tear, with virtually no generalized pain or swelling of his knee after a varus-contact injury, whose varsity coach designed plays for him so he did not need to cut, pivot, or twist to his left (affected) side. He was able to run, although much less effectively, within 1 week of injury. He did play an additional 2 weeks before it was recognized that he had a serious problem as his instability became more noticeable and his overall function worsened. I have found it best not to ask leading questions but rather to have patients describe their instability pattern in their own words. Frequently they report a "side-to-side toggling" of their knee, which helps me to recognize that they may have a posterolateral knee injury (**Fig. 4–2**).

I have found that patients with isolated posterolateral knee injuries do not complain of instability going down stairs or down hills, whereas patients who have concurrent posterior cruciate ligament tears often do complain of it. However, it has been demonstrated that the posterolateral knee structures do have some role in preventing primary posterior translation near extension,[6–8,12] so it is possible that a patient could complain of this problem in high-level activities involving descending.

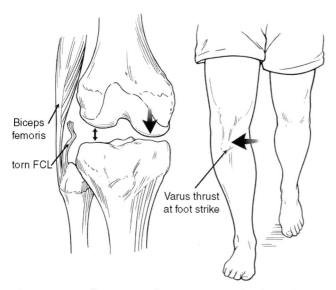

Biceps femoris

torn FCL

Varus thrust at foot strike

Figure 4–2 Illustration demonstrating the lateral compartment gapping (two-headed arrow) that can occur with a varus thrust (horizontal arrow) at foot strike in the face of a posterolateral knee injury. This can be accentuated by a weight-bearing mechanical axis through the medial compartment (vertical arrow).

References

1. Towne LC, Blazina ME, Marmor L, Lawrence JL. Lateral compartment syndrome of the knee. Clin Orthop Rel Res 1971;76:160–168

2. Hughston JC, Andrews JR, Cross MJ, Moschi A. Classification of knee ligament instabilities. Part II: the lateral compartment. J Bone Joint Surg 1976;58A:173–179

3. DeLee JC, Riley MB, Rockwood CA. Acute posterolateral rotatory instability of the knee. Am J Sports Med 1983;11:199–207

4. LaPrade RF, Terry GC. Injuries to the posterolateral aspect of the knee: association of anatomic injury patterns with clinical instability. Am J Sports Med 1997;25:433–438

5. Nielsen S, Rasmussen O, Ovesen J, Andersen K. Rotatory instability of cadaver knees after transaction of collateral ligaments and capsule. Arch Orthop Trauma Surg 1984;103:165–169

6. Gollehon DL, Torzilli PA, Warren RF. The role of the posterolateral and cruciate ligaments in the stability of the human knee: a biomechanical study. J Bone Joint Surg 1987;69A:233–242

7. Grood ES, Stowers SF, Noyes FR. Limits of movement in the human knee: effect of sectioning the posterior cruciate ligament and posterolateral structures. J Bone Joint Surg 1988;70A:88–97

8. Veltri DM, Deng X-H, Torzilli PA, Warren RF, Maynard MJ. The role of the cruciate and posterolateral ligaments in stability of the knee. Am J Sports Med 1995;23:436–443

9. Müller W. The Knee: Form, Function and Ligament Reconstruction. New York: Springer-Verlag, 1983

10. Baker CL, Norwood LA, Hughston JC. Acute combined posterior cruciate and posterolateral instability of the knee. Am J Sports Med 1983;11:308–314

11. Stäubli HU. Posteromedial and posterolateral capsular injuries associated with posterior cruciate ligament insufficiency. Sports Med Arthro Rev 1994;2:146–164

12. Veltri DM, Deng X-H, Torzilli PA, Maynard MJ, Warren RF. The role of the popliteofibular ligament in stability of the human knee: a biomechanical study. Am J Sports Med 1996;24:19–27

5

Clinical Examination of Posterolateral Knee Injuries

The portions of the physical examination that are useful for the diagnosis of posterolateral knee injuries are the external rotation recurvatum test, varus stress test at 30 degrees, dial test at 30 and 90 degrees, posterolateral drawer test, reverse pivot shift test, and an evaluation for a varus thrust gait.[1–8] Although many clinicians become skilled in the diagnosis of cruciate ligament injuries and develop a qualitative feel for knee laxity, the clinical examination assessment is still largely subjective, and its overall reliability depends on the skill and experience of the examiner. Because posterolateral knee injuries are commonly associated with other ligamentous injuries and may be missed at the time of the initial evaluation,[9–11] the injured knee should also be examined for ecchymosis, swelling, or tenderness over the posterolateral structures of the knee, especially for acute knee injuries. In addition, due to an approximate 15% incidence of associated common peroneal nerve injuries with posterolateral knee injuries, it is important to assess for the motor and sensory function of this nerve during the clinical examination of acute knee injuries.[11–13]

The external rotation recurvatum test assesses for increased genu recurvatum and relative genu varus[4] (Fig. 5–1). In this test, the patient lies supine on the examining table while the examiner lifts up the patient's great toe. It is important to compare the amount of recurvatum of the injured knee to the contralateral normal knee. A positive external rotation recurvatum test, where there is increased recurvatum and a relative varus position of the injured knee, usually indicates a combined cruciate ligament injury in addition to a posterolateral knee injury. In our experience, this usually means that a concurrent anterior cruciate ligament (ACL) tear is present.

The varus stress test is performed with the patient supine and the leg over the side of the examining table with the knee flexed to 30 degrees[1] (Fig. 5–2). A varus stress is applied to the knee through the foot/ankle, while the examiner's fingers palpate for the amount of lateral joint line opening. Due to physiologic

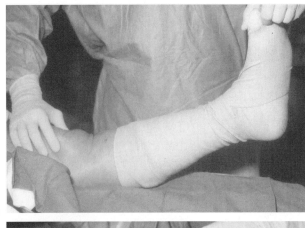

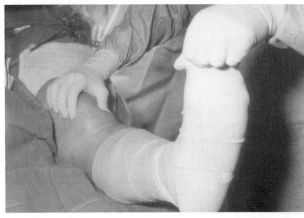

Figure 5–1   The external rotation recurvatum test. The examiner lifts the patient's great toe and assesses for an increased amount of knee recurvatum **(A)** and relative varus **(B)** compared with the normal contralateral knee. (From LaPrade RF, Terry GC. Injuries to the posterolateral aspect of the knee.

variations in the amount of normal lateral joint line opening, it is important to compare the amount of lateral joint line opening of the injured knee to the contralateral knee. The American Medical Association guidelines[14] for grade I (0–5 mm), grade II (6–10 mm), and grade III (>1 cm) joint line opening, compared with the normal contralateral knee, are followed to assess the severity of the posterolateral knee injury **(Table 5–1)**. It is important to recognize that increased varus opening will not be present without a concurrent injury to the fibular collateral ligament.[6,15–20]

The dial test assesses for an increased amount of external rotation of the tibia on the femur at 30 degrees **(Fig. 5–3)**. This test can be performed with the patient in either the supine or prone position; the amount of external rotation of the tibia compared with the femur in the injured knee is compared with that in the contralateral normal knee.[21,22] An external rotation force is applied to the

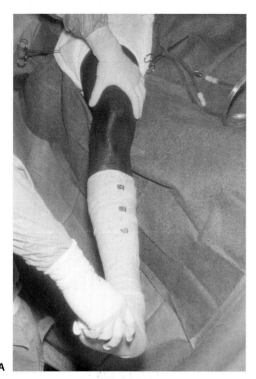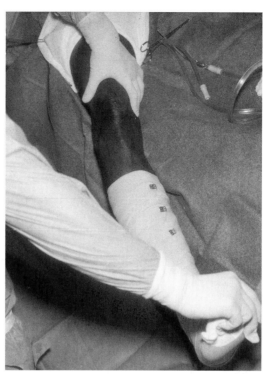

A   B

Figure 5–2 The varus stress test at 30 degrees. The examiner applies a varus force through the foot/ankle with one hand, while the other hand stabilizes the patient's knee and the examiner's fingers palpate to assess the amount of lateral joint-line opening. **(A)** Neutral position. **(B)** Varus force applied.

foot to determine the presence of increased rotation of the tibia on the femur compared with that in the normal contralateral knee. Visualization of the difference in rotation of the tibial tubercle is the best way to assess this study in the supine patient. Although this test has been found to be very specific in identifying posterolateral knee injuries in biomechanical sectioning studies,[6,18–20] it is a very subjective test that relies on subtleties in the physical examination. I believe that this makes the dial test one of the least useful tests clinically because it demonstrates relatively minor (10–15 degrees) visual changes in external rotation. In performing this test, it is very important to compare the increased external rotation of the injured knee to the normal contralateral knee. In a group of 30 normal volunteers who had their amount of tibial rotation calculated with a measurement device, the mean side-to-side difference between normal knees was 5.5 degrees at 30 degrees and 4.4 degrees at 90 degrees.[7] An increase in

Table 5–1   Classification of Varus Instability in Posterolateral Knee Injuries

AMA Grade	Amount of Varus Opening	Severity of Injury
I	0–5 mm	Mild
II	6–10 mm	Moderate
III	>1 cm	Severe

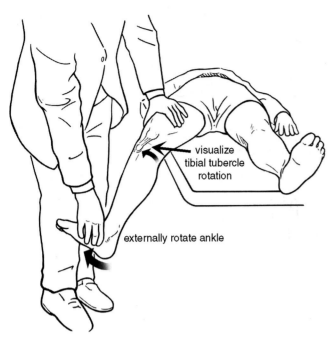

Figure 5–3   The dial test at 30 degrees of knee flexion. An external rotation force is applied to the knee and the amount of external rotation of the tibia, compared with the femur, is qualitatively measured by observing for differences in rotation of the tibial tubercles between the injured and normal contralateral knee.

external rotation of 10 to 15 degrees of the knee at 30 degrees is considered to be due to a posterolateral knee injury[6,19,20,23] **(Table 5–2)**.

In an isolated posterolateral knee injury, there should be a decrease in the amount of external rotation at 90 degrees compared with that found at 30 degrees.[6,20,24] The amount of increased external rotation seen at 90 degrees of knee flexion compared with the contralateral normal knee with an isolated posterolateral knee injury should be 5 to 7 degrees.[20,25] However, if there is a concurrent posterior cruciate ligament (PCL) tear, there will be an increase in external rotation at 90 degrees.[20,26] In addition, with a concurrent ACL tear, there also appears to be a similar increase in external rotation at 90 degrees with a combined posterolateral knee injury, which averages 15 degrees compared with the contralateral normal knee.[27] Therefore, an increase of external

Table 5–2   Classification of External Rotation Increases at 30 Degrees in Posterolateral Knee Injuries

Grade	Degrees of Increased External Rotation	Severity of Injury
I	0–5 degrees	Mild
II	6–10 degrees	Moderate
III	>10 degrees	Severe

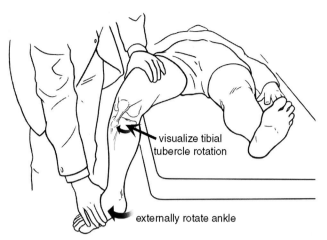

Figure 5–4   The dial test at 90 degrees. An external rotation force is applied to the foot/ankle and the amount of rotation of the tibial tubercle is observed. For an isolated posterolateral knee injury, the amount of increased external rotation averages between 5 and 7 degrees. An increase in external rotation to between 10 and 15 degrees would indicate a probable concurrent posterior or anterior cruciate ligament tear and a combined posterolateral knee injury.

rotation clinically seen on the dial test at 90 degrees of knee flexion can be due to either a concurrent ACL or PCL injury **(Fig. 5–4)**.

The posterolateral drawer test[4] is performed at 90 degrees of knee flexion with the foot externally rotated 15 degrees **(Fig. 5–5)**. A posterolateral force is applied to the knee to assess for an increase in knee joint motion. An increase in a combined, coupled posterolateral rotation compared with the normal contralateral knee is indicative of a posterolateral knee injury. It is important clinically to

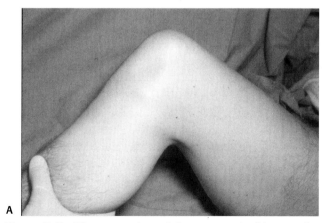
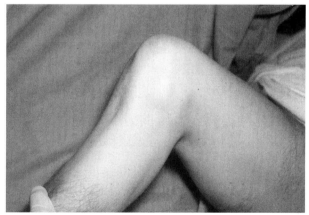

A   **B**

Figure 5–5   The posterolateral drawer test. In this test, the knee is flexed to 90 degrees and the foot is externally rotated to 15 degrees. The examiner applies a gentle posterolateral rotation force to the knee and the amount of posterolateral rotation of the tibia on the femur is qualitatively measured compared with the normal contralateral knee. **(A)** Neutral position. **(B)** Posterolateral drawer applied.

Table 5–3 Classification of Posterolateral Knee Injuries

Grade	Sprain Type	Clinical Findings
Grade I	Minor sprain	Minimal increase in varus translation, external rotation at 30 and 90 degrees, and posterolateral drawer at 90 degrees
Grade II	Moderate sprain	An increase of varus less than 1 cm (compared with the contralateral side) with a palpable end point; an increase of external rotation at 30 degrees less than 10 degrees; an increase in posterolateral drawer no more than one grade compared with the contralateral side
Grade III	Severe sprain	Greater than 1 cm of varus opening at 30 degrees; a 10-degree increase of external rotation at 30 degrees compared with the contralateral side; a one to two grade increase in the posterolateral drawer test at 90 degrees compared with the contralateral side

differentiate this test from the posterior drawer test in neutral rotation, which primarily assesses the integrity of the posterior cruciate ligament[4] (**Table 5–3**).

The reverse pivot shift test[5] is a dynamic test to assess for posterolateral rotation of the tibia on the femur (**Fig. 5–6**). I consider it to be a dynamic variant of the posterolateral drawer test. This test has been noted to have the most variability of all motion tests and has been found to be positive in 35% of normal

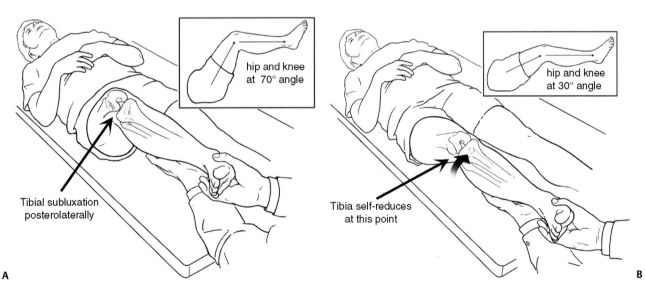

Figure 5–6 The reverse pivot shift test. **(A)** The knee is flexed to between 70 and 90 degrees and the foot is externally rotated, which would result in posterolateral subluxation of the tibia on the femur. **(B)** The knee is then extended while the knee is observed for a reduction of the posterolaterally subluxed tibia on the femur at about 30 degrees.

knees examined under anesthesia.[21] In this test, the knee is flexed to 70 to 90 degrees and the foot is externally rotated. The knee is then slowly extended and observed to see if a reduction of a posterolaterally subluxed tibia occurs on the femur. The reverse pivot shift test is considered to be positive when a noticeable reduction of the tibia occurs on the femur. Due to the large physiologic variability among patients with a normal knee and a positive reverse pivot shift test, especially in patients with physiologic genu recurvatum, the test leg itself is rarely useful to determine the presence of a posterolateral knee injury in isolation.

Tears of the popliteomeniscal fascicles can result in lateral meniscal hypermobility and entrapment of the lateral meniscus in the joint with application of a varus stress. Patients who present with this pathology often complain of vague lateral joint knee pain, and MRI scans are often inconclusive. In these patients, the figure-four test, where the ipsilateral foot is placed over the contralateral knee, has been found to be an accurate method to diagnose popliteomeniscal fascicle tears with resulting lateral meniscal entrapment.[28]

In addition to these clinical tests specific for the assessment of posterolateral knee injuries, it is important to assess for increased amounts of anterior tibial translation on the Lachman test. The increased posterior translation seen at 30 degrees with a posterolateral knee injury,[6,20,24] as well as the increase in anterior translation seen with posterolateral structure injury in the face of a concurrent ACL tear,[19,24,27] may be detected clinically as increased anterior translation in both an ACL-intact (a "pseudo-Lachman" test) and ACL-deficient knee with the Lachman test. If there is a solid end point present (in an ACL-intact knee) with increased anterior translation on the Lachman test, one should be suspicious of a possible underlying posterolateral knee injury with its associated increase in posterior translation in early flexion.[6,20,24,29] Thus, a positive pseudo-Lachman test may be positive with either a concurrent PCL or posterolateral knee injury (or both). It is also important to recognize that a significant increase in anterior translation in an ACL-deficient knee on the Lachman test of the injured knee may signify an underlying posterolateral knee injury. In those knees that have an ACL tear, a 3+ or 4+ Lachman test, and an intact PCL and posterior horn of the medial meniscus, one should assume that a posterolateral knee injury has to be ruled out of the clinical diagnosis.

In addition, posterior translation of the knee in neutral rotation should be carefully assessed. If posterior translation of the knee is slightly increased at 30 degrees, but near normal at 90 degrees (with a negative or trace positive quadriceps active test),[30] then a posterolateral knee injury (with an intact PCL) should be suspected. If posterior knee translation in neutral rotation at 90 degrees is also significantly increased, then in addition to a PCL injury, a combined posterolateral corner injury should also be suspected.[6,20] It is becoming increasingly recognized that most isolated PCL tears result in <1 cm of increased posterior translation with a clinical posterior drawer test of 1+ to 2+. In a knee with a 3+ posterior drawer test or for which ≥12 mm of increased posterior translation is seen on stress radiographs, one must rule out a combined posterolateral and PCL tear.

In addition to these clinical tests for abnormal joint motion, it is also important to assess for any potential motor or sensory deficits of the common peroneal nerve. This would include an assessment of sensation in the first dorsal web space and dorsal and lateral aspect of the foot and an assessment of motor strength of the extensor hallucis longus, extensor digitorum longus, and ankle dorsiflexors and evertors.

Finally, a patient should be assessed for the presence of a varus-thrust gait with ambulation.[8,31–33] In patients with this gait abnormally, a varus thrusting occurs due to a high adduction moment as the ligamentous-deficient lateral compartment opens up at foot strike during the stance phase of the gait cycle. With further ambulation, the dynamic action of the biceps femoris and a shift of the center of gravity of the body with a forward gait stride help to close down the increased varus opening of the lateral compartment. As it closes down, a visible shift (thrust) of the affected knee is seen. Patients can sometimes adapt and prevent this gait abnormality by ambulating with a flexed knee gait,[33] which helps to decrease abnormal lateral compartment opening in a posterolateral deficient knee. Although most of these patients have an underlying varus alignment of their knees that contributes to this instability, not all patients have an underlying genu varus alignment.

◆ Radiographic Evaluation of Posterolateral Knee Injuries

Plain radiographs of a knee with a posterolateral knee injury may show a Segond fracture[34] (**Fig. 5–7**), arcuate fracture[35] (**Fig. 5–8**), or abnormal widening of the lateral compartment joint space.[8] In addition, patients with chronic

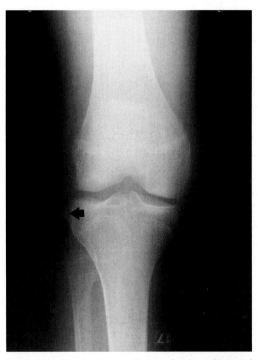

Figure 5–7 Anteroposterior (AP) radiograph demonstrating a Segond avulsion fracture (arrow) of the meniscotibial portion of the mid-third lateral capsular ligament and the anterior arm of the short head of the biceps femoris off the tibia (right knee).

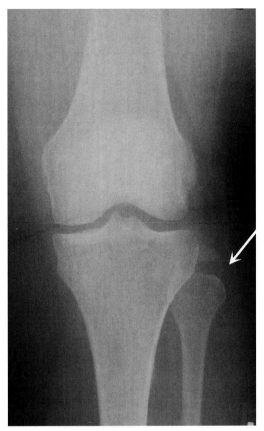

Figure 5–8. An AP radiograph demonstrating an "arcuate" avulsion fracture of the fibular styloid (left knee).

posterolateral knee injuries may have degenerative changes of the medial compartment.[3,36] Anteroposterior (AP) varus-thrust radiographs have also been noted to be helpful in demonstrating the amount of increased lateral joint line opening, but are not routinely done as part of initial radiographic screening[8] **(Fig. 5–9)**.

Other radiographs that can be useful to assess the extent of a posterolateral corner injury include bilateral PCL stress radiographs. It has been noted that isolated complete PCL tears usually have an 8- to 10-mm side-to-side difference in posterior knee translation on stress radiographs. In these cases in which the amount of posterior translation increases to >12 mm, then one should suspect a probable concurrent posterolateral (or potential posteromedial) knee injury **(Fig. 5–10)**.

Although a Segond fracture[34] has been described to be pathognomonic for an ACL tear,[37] it has also been noted to be present in the face of posterolateral knee injuries.[11,38] Originally described to be an avulsion of a fleck of bone off the proximolateral tibia with its attached lateral capsule,[34,37,39] it has since been found frequently to have also the anterior arm of the short head of the biceps femoris attached to the avulsed tissues.[40] I have found in some instances that Segond fractures, or Segond soft tissue avulsion injury variants, are much larger

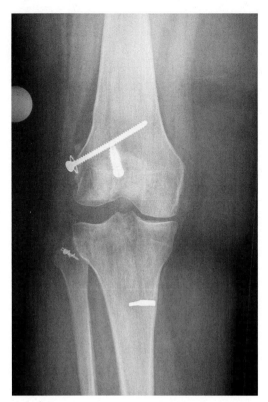

Figure 5–9 An AP standing varus-thrust radiograph demonstrating increased lateral compartment gapping in the face of a posterolateral knee injury (right knee).

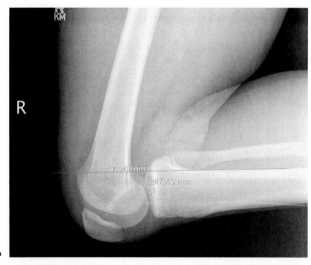
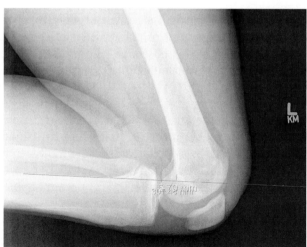

Figure 5–10 Bilateral posterior cruciate ligament (PCL) stress radiographs. The reference points include a parallel line drawn along the posterior crest of the tibial and a point indicating the posterior aspect of Blumensaat's line. A posterior translation of greater than 12 mm is indicative of a combined posterior cruciate ligament and probable posterolateral (or posteromedial) knee injury. **(A)** Injured knee. **(B)** Normal knee. There is a 22-mm difference in this combined PCL and posterolateral knee injury.

and sometimes contain the entire lateral capsular attachments in the face of a posterolateral knee injury.

Platt[12] and Watson-Jones[13] reported on avulsion fractures of the fibular head or styloid associated with lateral-based knee injuries and concurrent common peroneal nerve injuries. DeLee et al[41] noted the presence of a fibular head fracture in five of 12 patients with acute posterolateral rotatory instability treated surgically. They concluded that x-ray evidence of a fibular head avulsion suggests the presence of a lateral ligament injury. Shindell et al[35] were the first to describe an avulsion fracture of the fibular head and styloid as an "arcuate" fracture. They reported that it represented an avulsion of bone with the fibular collateral ligament and other structures (popliteofibular ligament, fabellofibular ligament, and capsular arm of the short head of the biceps femoris) attached to the fibular head, and that this fracture was indicative of a posterolateral corner knee injury.

In addition to the standard AP and lateral radiographs of the knee, it is important to obtain full-length standing AP (hip to ankle) radiographs in patients with chronic posterolateral knee injuries to assess for the presence of genu varus alignment of the lower extremity **(Fig. 5–11)**. Failure to correct genu varus alignment prior to repair/reconstruction of chronic posterolateral knee injuries has been associated with stretching out of posterolateral repairs or reconstructions.[8,33,42,43]

Varus Thrust Standing Anteroposterior or Varus Stress Radiographs

It is well recognized in a clinical situation that it can be very difficult to determine the neutral axis point in a patient who may have a combined medial collateral ligament complex injury, significant physiologic varus opening, or medial compartment pseudolaxity due to medial compartment arthritic changes. In spite of an astute ability to pick up the amount of lateral compartment opening in most patients, one may find that in some patients the amount of lateral compartment opening cannot be sufficiently assessed to be able to arrive at a judgment of the severity of a potential posterolateral corner injury. In these circumstances, I have found that the addition of varus thrust standing AP or varus stress radiographs to be very effective in delineating the extent of lateral compartment opening.

Varus stress standing AP radiographs are obtained with the patient standing and attempting to thrust the lateral compartment open. The difference in lateral compartment opening in the thrust radiograph is then compared with the standing AP radiograph to determine if the patient is having clinical instability due to lateral compartment gapping.

Varus stress AP radiographs are obtained on both knees to help determine the amount of lateral compartment opening on the affected side compared with the contralateral normal knee. It is very important to make sure that these radiographs are obtained in about 15 to 20 degrees of knee flexion, that the same amount of stress is relatively applied to each knee by the examiner, and that there is no rotation of the radiographs, which could throw off the measurements **(Fig. 5–12)**. To do these radiographs, the examiner will place a lead shielded hand along the patient's thigh while the other hand is used to apply the varus

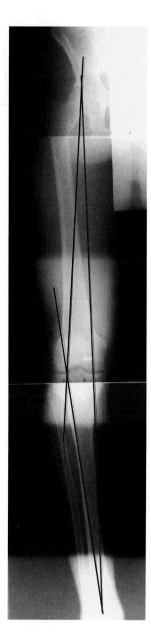

Figure 5–11 Full length, hip-to-ankle, standing radiograph of the right lower extremity to assess lower extremity alignment. The mechanical axis is calculated from a line drawn from the center of the femoral head to the center of the ankle for a normal mechanical axis. This line should pass through the center of the knee. Genu varus is present for any mechanical axis that is medial to the tip of the medial tibial spine.

stress to the knee through the distal foot or ankle. It is important to coordinate the application of the varus stress with the radiology technician taking the radiographs, so that the patient does not have reflex guarding, which could potentially decrease the amount of lateral compartment opening as the dynamic function of the biceps femoris helps to close down the lateral compartment gapping. In addition, if there is some concern about a possible concurrent medial-sided knee injury, valgus stress radiographs may also be performed at this time. It is important to recognize this injury as a potential source of symptoms due to the fact that injuries to the posterior oblique ligament can result in relative increases of external rotation of the tibia on the femur due to the anteromedial instability

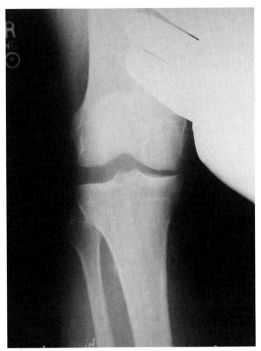

Figure 5–12 An AP varus stress radiograph demonstrating increased lateral compartment opening in a knee with a posterolateral corner injury (right knee).

pattern created. Thus, if one does not recognize the side-to-side toggle as occurring from the medial compartment, rather than the lateral compartment, it may be believed that the increase in external rotation and the side-to-side toggle of the knee is due to a posterolateral corner injury when, in fact, it may be due to a posteromedial ligament injury.

◆ Magnetic Resonance Imaging of Posterolateral Knee Injuries

Hassine et al[44] reported on the MRI appearance of the popliteal hiatus and the structures that coursed from the fibula to the posterolateral corner of the knee with correlations to cadaveric knee cross-sectional anatomy dissections (four knees), and also for both normal and injured patients' knees. In this study, which was performed using a 0.5-tesla (low strength) MRI magnet, the authors described the MRI appearance of the normal popliteus tendon and surrounding structures and demonstrated that tears of these structures, verified by open or arthroscopic surgical treatment, could be identified on MRI scans.

Ruiz and Erickson[45] reported on the MRI appearance of some normal posterolateral knee structures (on a 1.5-tesla MRI unit) and injured structures (on a 0.5-tesla MRI unit) according to Seebacher et al's[46] three-layered description of posterolateral knee anatomy. In this pictorial description of MRI findings, they reported on the MRI appearance of the fibular collateral ligament, inferior lateral genicular vessels, biceps femoris, common peroneal nerve, lateral gastrocnemius tendon, popliteus tendon, iliotibial band, and Segond and fibular head avulsion fractures.

Tardieu et al[47] reported on a retrospective study on a 0.5-tesla (low-resolution MRI) magnet of a group of selected patients with posterolateral knee injuries who had surgical correlation with the MRI readings. The MRI appearances of several posterolateral structures were presented. Brown et al[48] reported on the MRI appearance of popliteus complex injuries in a group of 24 patients taken from 2412 consecutive knee MRIs (~1% of MRIs) performed on a 1.5-tesla MRI unit with an extremity coil. The authors felt that 23 of 24 of the patients with popliteus complex injuries had tears of the muscle belly (as evidenced by enlargement of the muscle and high signal intensity on T2-weighted images) and only one patient was found to have an isolated tear of the popliteus tendon on MRI. No clinical correlation or confirmation was provided for this group of patients.

Yu et al[49] reported on a coronal oblique imaging technique that was aligned parallel to the course of the popliteus tendon utilizing a 1.5-tesla (high-resolution) magnet. They followed a prospective group of 100 patients to determine if they could image the fabellofibular ligament, "arcuate" ligament (i.e., the capsular arm of the short head of the biceps femoris), fibular origin of the popliteal muscle (i.e., the popliteofibular ligament), fibular collateral ligament, and biceps femoris tendon. They found that the addition of the coronal oblique imaging plane improved visualization compared with the standard coronal plane for the arcuate ligament (i.e., the short head of the biceps femoris) (46% vs. 10% visualized, respectively), fabellofibular ligament (48% vs. 34% visualized), and fibular origin of the popliteal muscle (i.e., the popliteofibular ligament) (53% vs. 8% visualized). They recommended the addition of coronal oblique T2-weighted images to the MRI protocols of patients with suspected posterolateral knee injuries. However, because their study did not include patients with posterolateral knee injuries, the ability of this technique to recognize injuries was not investigated. In addition, no surgical correlation was noted for their imaging findings. A critical review of this study reveals that the authors called the lateral gastrocnemius tendon the fabellofibular ligament in one of their sagittal images (**Fig. 5–13**).

Ross et al[50] reported on the MRI appearance of six consecutive patients with acute posterolateral knee injuries who also had concurrent ACL tears. Four of these patients underwent an open repair of their posterolateral knee injuries. Magnetic resonance imaging was found to be accurate in these four patients in diagnosing injuries to the iliotibial band, biceps femoris tendon, popliteus tendon, and the fibular collateral ligament.

Miller et al[51] performed anatomic dissections on cadaveric knees and painted the fibular collateral ligament, popliteus tendon, and popliteofibular ligament with barium. Radiographs were then obtained of these anatomic specimens to demonstrate their course on plain radiographs to assist with the interpretation of MRI scans. The authors then retrospectively reviewed the reports of 481 MRI scans obtained at their institution and found 30 cases in which posterolateral knee injuries had been identified (6% of cases). They reported

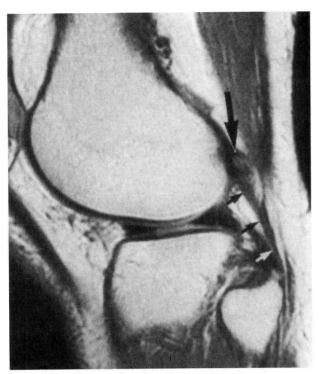

Figure 5–13 This sagittal magnetic resonance imaging (MRI) scan demonstrates that the coronal course of a lateral gastrocnemius tendon (not the fabellofibular ligament as reported in Yu et al[49]). Long arrow, fabella; short arrows, lateral gastrochemius tendon. (From Yu JS, Salonen DC, Hodler J, Haghighi P, Trudell D, Resnick D. Posterolateral aspect of the knee: improved MR imaging with a coronal oblique technique. Radiology 1996;198:199–204, with permission.)

that 19 fibular collateral ligament tears, 16 popliteus musculotendinous injuries, and three biceps femoris tendon injuries were identified in this group of patients. They concluded that MRI was capable of identifying posterolateral knee injuries in light of the fact only three of these 30 patients had suspected posterolateral knee injuries prior to the MRI scan. The total clinical incidence of posterolateral knee injuries in this group of patients is unknown.

Because of the lack of clear information in the literature describing the MRI diagnosis of posterolateral knee injuries, I found that many referred patients with posterolateral knee injuries had inconclusive MRI scans for posterolateral knee injuries due to a failure either to include the entire fibular head and styloid on the MRI scans, or to have thick-sliced scans (4 mm or larger); thus the scans missed many of the posterolateral knee structures.

For this reason, we then performed a study looking at normal knees and the injured appearance of posterolateral knee injuries.[52] We were able to demonstrate that the MRI protocol that was developed yielded accurate visualization of the majority of the complex individual anatomic components of the posterolateral knee.

We found that this imaging protocol, which included the entire fibular head and styloid, using thin slices (2 mm), a high-resolution scanner (1.5-tesla or potentially higher resolution), and coronal oblique views placed in line with the course of the popliteus tendon (**Fig. 5–14**) provided a useful adjunct to the diagnosis of posterolateral knee injuries. In addition, the MRI scans were found to assist the surgeon in the preoperative planning of surgical incisions and in determining whether a repair or reconstruction of an injured structure was necessary (**Fig. 5–15**). For example, some injuries to individual structures of the posterolateral knee can be very difficult to repair[38] and may need a reconstruction with autografts or allografts (which is useful information to know prior to a surgical procedure). In particular, midsubstance fibular collateral ligament tears, popliteus musculotendinous avulsions, and midsubstance popliteus tendon tears are very difficult to repair in the acutely injured knee.[38] In these instances, and for chronic posterolateral knee injuries, where structures are attenuated or retracted and encased in scar tissue, the surgeon may need to consider a surgical reconstruction rather than an attempted repair of these structures. It is very useful to know this information preoperatively so the correct surgical instruments or ligament allografts can be obtained prior to surgery.

In addition, we identified the presence of a soft tissue avulsion, with the same structures avulsed that have been noted to be attached to a bony Segond fracture avulsion (anterior arm of the short head of the biceps femoris and meniscotibial portion of the mid-third lateral capsular ligament); this avulsion was commonly found in the presence of a posterolateral knee injury. We have termed this a "soft tissue Segond avulsion" pattern. Like the bony Segond fracture, it is a nonspecific MRI finding for posterolateral knee injuries, and we hypothesize it may commonly be found in the face of an ACL tear.

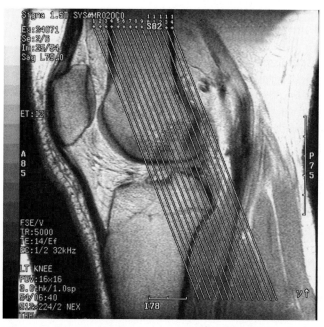

Figure 5–14   Coronal oblique scout MRI sagittal film demonstrating that the coronal oblique view is placed in line with the intraarticular course of the popliteus tendon over the posterolateral aspect of the knee (left knee).

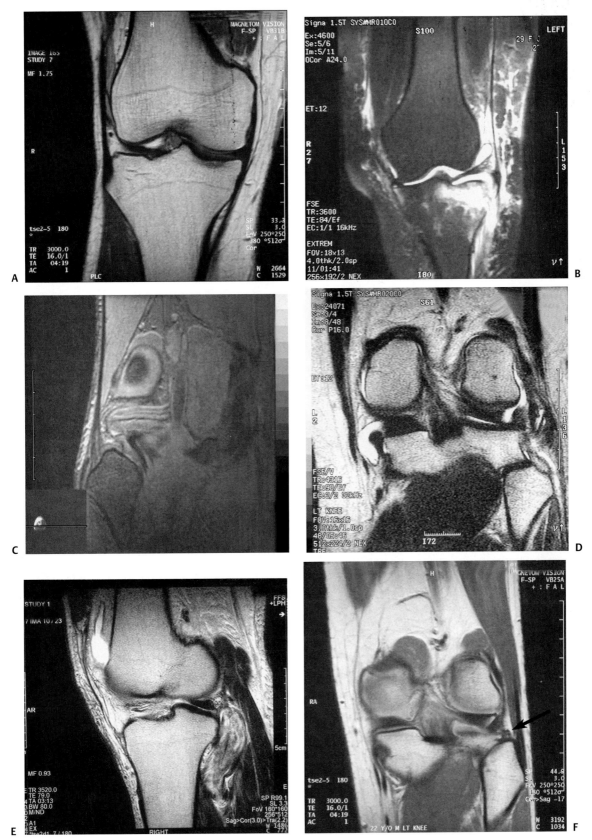

Figure 5–15

(*Continued on page 96*)

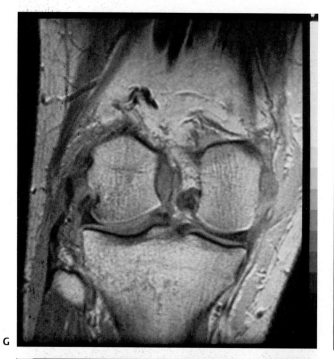

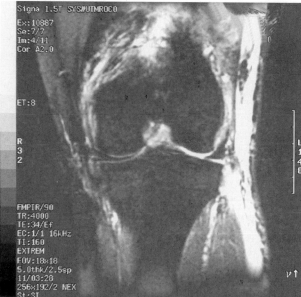

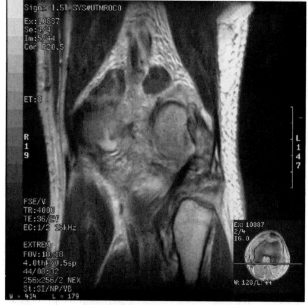

Figure 5–15 (*Continued*)   Coronal MRI scans of normal and injured posterolateral knee structures. **(A)** Normal iliotibial band (right knee). **(B)** Avulsion of iliotibial band off Gerdy's tubercle (left knee). **(C)** Normal attachment of direct arms of the long and short heads of the biceps femoris on the fibular styloid (right knee). **(D)** Avulsed biceps femoris structures off fibular styloid (left knee). **(E)** Sagittal MRI scan demonstrating the typical popliteus muscle belly edema seen in an acute popliteus musculotendinous junction injury (right knee). **(F)** Torn popliteofibular ligament (left knee). **(G)** Coronal MRI scan (right knee) demonstrating a tear of the fibular collateral ligament off the femur. **(H)** Soft tissue Segond avulsion off tibia with mid-third lateral capsular ligament and anterior arm of the short head of the biceps femoris avulsed (left knee). **(I)** "Arcuate" avulsion fracture with biceps femoris components and popliteofibular ligament attached (left knee).

Electromyelogram or Nerve Conduction Velocity Studies

There may be times where it is necessary in the face of posterolateral corner knee injuries to include electromyelogram (EMG)/nerve conduction velocity (NCV) studies to determine either the integrity of the common peroneal nerve as it crosses the fibular head, or to determine if there is a significant neuropraxia of the nerve with scar tissue entrapment. I have not found these tests to be very useful in the majority of patients, but it is recognized that there may be times when these tests would be appropriate. I have found them to be useful in patients who sustain a contusion to the posterolateral corner of the knee and have continued residual posterolateral knee pain without any evidence of objective laxity. In those patients who are found to have irritation of the common peroneal nerve to palpation, along its course just posterior to the long head of the biceps and before it crosses under the peroneus longus fascia, it may be appropriate to obtain an EMG/NCV study to determine if there is any entrapment of the nerve in this location. In those circumstances in which there does appear to be some entrapment of the common peroneal nerve at this location, I have performed an open peroneal nerve neurolysis, about two or three times a year, with a vast majority of patients noting a significant improvement of their subjective pain and dysesthesia symptoms due to the common peroneal nerve entrapment at this location.

◆ Arthroscopic Evaluation of the Lateral Component of Knees with Grade 3 Posterolateral Knee Complex Injuries

Arthroscopic evaluation of the lateral compartment of knees with posterolateral knee injuries has been found to be effective in the identification of the majority of injuries to the popliteus complex (popliteus femoral attachment, popliteus tendon, and popliteomeniscal fascicles) (**Fig. 5–16**), coronary ligament to the

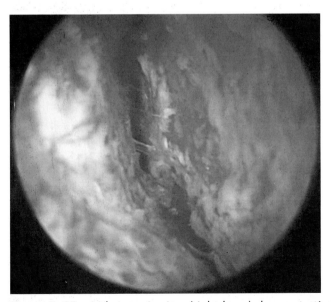

Figure 5–16 Arthroscopic view (right knee) demonstrating a tear of the popliteus tendon off its femoral attachment.

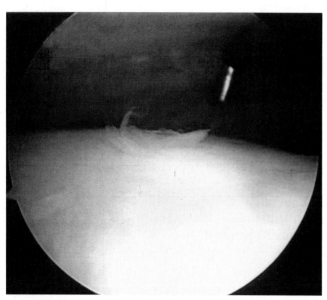

Figure 5–17   Arthroscopic view (right knee) demonstrating a tear of the coronary ligament of the posterior horn of the lateral meniscus.

lateral meniscus (**Fig. 5–17**), lateral meniscus, and the meniscofemoral and meniscotibial portions of the mid-third lateral capsular ligament.[53,54] Visualization of the popliteomeniscal fascicles and popliteofibular ligament was performed with the arthroscope in the lateral gutter with the knee in about 20 degrees of knee flexion and a slight valgus force applied. However, analysis of the integrity of the popliteofibular ligament by arthroscopic evaluation was not successful in the majority of patients who were found to have an injury to this structure during an open repair. Stäubli and Birrer[55] also noted difficulty in visualizing the popliteofibular ligament arthroscopically. This discrepancy may be explained by the fact that only the more proximal aspect of the anterior division of the popliteofibular ligament was able to be visualized arthroscopically and not its main portion that attaches to the posteromedial aspect of the fibular styloid. In addition, in those patients with a proximal avulsion of the popliteus tendon off the femur (33%), distal migration of the popliteus tendon and resultant scar tissue, hematoma, or synovitis in the popliteal hiatus made it difficult to visualize the popliteofibular ligament arthroscopically. I believe that it is possible that the addition of a 70-degree arthroscope, to supplement the findings seen with the standard 30-degree arthroscope, could allow for improved visualization of the normal and injured popliteofibular ligament by arthroscopic evaluation. Clinically, one needs to place the arthroscope deep into the popliteal hiatus with the knee flexed to about 20 to 25 degrees and a slight valgus force applied to the knee so the lateral compartment is not closed down. One can then rotate the arthroscope while it is in this gap and follow the distal fibers of the anteroinferior popliteomeniscal fascicle, which blends at its distal margin with the anterior division of the popliteofibular ligament, to arthroscopically assess for a possible tear of the popliteofibular ligament.

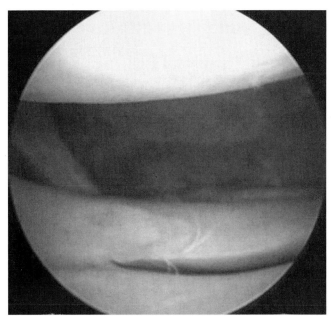

Figure 5–18 Arthroscopic "drive-through" sign of the lateral compartment of greater than 1 cm of opening consistent with a posterolateral knee injury (right knee).

All 30 knees in this study had greater than 1 cm of lateral compartment joint opening with application of a varus stress to the knee as measured with a surgical probe. This has been termed the "drive-through" sign[53] (**Fig. 5–18**). It is recommended that if this sign is encountered in a patient with an unsuspected posterolateral knee ligamentous injury, the knee should be reexamined, either arthroscopically or with a repeat examination under anesthesia (EUA), to rule out a posterolateral knee injury because the implications of a missed, or ignored, posterolateral knee injury on a patient's long-term function or in the face of a concurrent cruciate ligament reconstruction can be significant.[33,38,56,57]

Overall, the arthroscopic evaluation of the lateral compartment of knees with grade 3 posterolateral knee injuries revealed a significant number of pathologic changes that may have gone undetected if only an open reconstruction had been performed. Arthroscopic evaluation of the knee helped to facilitate the placement of surgical incisions by enhancing visualization of specific intraarticular structures. The arthroscopic evaluation of the lateral compartment assisted with the decision on whether a lateral capsular arthrotomy incision was necessary (to address popliteus tendon avulsions or injuries, popliteomeniscal fascicle tears with an unstable lateral meniscus to surgical probing, or other lateral-sided intraarticular pathology) or if a dissection to access the posterior knee, which would be a further development of the interval between the soleus and lateral gastrocnemius muscles, was necessary to repair injuries to the coronary ligament (meniscotibial portion of the posterior capsule) of the posterior horn of the lateral meniscus. In addition, the arthroscopic evaluation can assist with the determination of whether

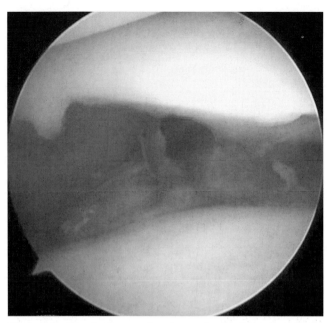

Figure 5–19 Arthroscopic view of the lateral compartment of a right knee demonstrating a meniscotibial-based avulsion injury pattern.

the meniscus is stable and attached to the tibia (with a meniscofemoral-based injury) or if its meniscotibial attachments are torn **(Fig. 5–19)**.

◆ Differential Diagnosis to Posterolateral Knee Injuries

The clinical diagnosis of posterolateral knee injuries can sometimes be confused with other etiologies of presumed increases in clinical motion testing. It is recognized that in some instances the amount of measured laxity may present similarly to posterolateral instability from injuries.

Patients who have advanced medial compartment arthritis, especially in those who have a genu varus alignment, may present with lateral compartment "pseudolaxity" to varus stressing at 30 degrees of knee flexion due to medial compartment collapse from a lack of articular cartilage of the medial joint compartment. Similarly, these patients often may have a varus-thrust gait with ambulation for the same reasons. In addition to the patient's history, AP standing and long leg alignment radiographs are necessary to assist in the proper diagnosis in this instance.

Another condition that may present as a possible case of posterolateral knee instability is acute or chronic anteromedial rotatory instability of the knee. I have had patients referred to me with a diagnosis of posterolateral rotatory instability who were found on physical exam to have an increase in external rotation laxity but in fact were found to have either an acute or chronic tear of the superficial medial collateral ligament and a combined posterior oblique ligament tear. In these instances, there was an increase in anteromedial rotatory instability that at first appeared to be due to an increase in external rotation of the tibia on the femur. In these cases, the clinical exam, and often valgus stress radiographs (to confirm my diagnosis and contradict the referring diagnosis), demonstrated that the medial to lateral toggle of the knee felt at 30 degrees of knee flexion was in fact due to an increase in the medial compartment, rather than lateral compartment, joint line opening.

◆ Conclusion

It has been well recognized that in spite of an increasing number of publications over the past decade that have better defined the anatomy, diagnosis, and treatment of injuries to the posterolateral knee, posterolateral rotatory instability of the knee is still difficult to diagnose clinically. This is especially true in the acute situation because significant protective guarding may make it difficult for the patient to sufficiently relax for the clinician to determine the extent of a posterolateral knee injury. In addition, in light of an obvious ACL or PCL injury, a posterolateral knee injury may not be recognized by the clinician. It is commonly necessary to combine several of the clinical motion tests (external rotation recurvatum test, varus stress test at 30 degrees, dial test at 30 and 90 degrees, posterolateral drawer test, reverse pivot shift test, evaluation for a varus thrust gait, and increases in translation for the Lachman test or posterior drawer test) to determine the extent of a posterolateral knee injury. In spite of this, guarding by the patient or combined ligament injuries, where it is difficult to determine the normal position of the knee, may make it very difficult to determine the extent of a posterolateral knee injury. Also, a large number of patients have increased physiologic posterolateral knee laxity,[21] which can make it difficult to determine if the patient has physiologic laxity or a possible injury to the posterolateral knee when there is a concurrent cruciate ligament tear. In light of the difficulty in arriving at a diagnosis of a acute or chronic posterolateral corner injury, an attempt has been made to develop additional means of diagnosing posterolateral corner injuries to aid the clinician in assessing these debilitating injuries when the diagnosis may be in doubt. The addition of plain knee radiographs, varus or posterior stress radiographs, and MRI scans with specific cuts has been found to be useful to aid the clinician in the diagnosis of these difficult injuries.

In addition, even an adequately performed exam under anesthesia may not confirm whether a patient has a posterolateral knee injury, especially if the contralateral knee has a component of physiologic posterolateral knee laxity. In this instance, the addition of a diagnostic arthroscopic evaluation has been found to be very useful to aid in the diagnosis of posterolateral knee injuries and to assist in the evaluation of surgical incisions to address posterolateral knee injuries. Identification of an arthroscopic drive-through sign of greater than 1 cm of increased lateral joint line opening of the lateral compartment with application of a varus stress should enable one clinically to rule out a posterolateral knee injury.

References

1. Hughston JC. Knee ligament injuries in athletes. Med J Ala 1966;36:243–252
2. Hughston JC, Andrews JR, Cross MJ, Moschi A. Classification of knee ligament injuries. Part I: the medial compartment and cruciate ligaments. J Bone Joint Surg 1976;58A:159–172
3. Hughston JC, Andrews JR, Cross MJ, Moschi A. Classification of knee ligament instabilities. Part II: the lateral compartment. J Bone Joint Surg 1976B;58A:173–179
4. Hughston JC, Norwood LA. The posterolateral drawer test and external rotation recurvation test for posterolateral rotatory instability of the knee. Clin Ortho Rel Res 1980;147:82–87
5. Jakob RP, Hassler H, Stäubli HU. Observations on rotatory instability of the lateral compartment of the knee: experimental studies on the functional anatomy and pathomechanism of the true and reversed pivot shift sign. Acta Orthop Scand Suppl 1981;191:1–32
6. Gollehon DL, Torzilli PA, Warren RF. The role of the posterolateral and cruciate ligaments in the stability of the human knee: a biomechanical study. J Bone Joint Surg 1987;69A:233–242
7. Bleday RM, Fanelli GC, Glannotti BF, Edson CJ, Barrett TA. Instrumented measurement of the posterolateral corner. Arthroscopy 1998;14:489–494
8. LaPrade RF. The medial collateral ligament complex and posterolateral aspect of the knee. In: Sports Medicine Orthopaedic Knowledge Update (OKU). Chicago: American Academy of Orthopaedic Surgeons, 1999
9. Baker CL, Norwood LA, Hughston JC. Acute combined posterior cruciate and posterolateral instability of the knee. Am J Sports Med 1983;11:308–314
10. DeLee JC, Riley MB, Rockwood CA. Acute posterolateral rotatory instability of the knee. Am J Sports Med 1983;11:199–207
11. LaPrade RF, Terry GC. Injuries to the posterolateral aspect of the knee: association of anatomic injury patterns with clinical instability. Am J Sports Med 1997;25:433–438
12. Platt H. On the peripheral nerve complications of certain fractures. J Bone Joint Surg 1928;10:403–414
13. Watson-Jones R. Styloid process of fibula in the knee joint with peroneal palsy. J Bone Joint Surg 1931;13:258–260
14. American Medical Association (AMA). Standard Nomenclature of Athletic Injuries. Chicago: American Medical Association, 1966
15. Markolf KL, Mensch JS, Amstutz H. Stiffness and laxity of the knee—the contributions of the supporting structures. J Bone Joint Surg 1976;58A:583–594
16. Seering WP, Piziali RL, Nagel DA, Schurman DJ. The function of the primary ligaments of the knee in varus-valgus and axial rotation. J Biomech 1980;13:785–794
17. Grood ES, Noyes FR, Butler DL, Suntay WJ. Ligamentous and capsular restraints preventing straight medial and lateral laxity in intact human cadaver knees. J Bone Joint Surg 1981;63A:1257–1269
18. Nielsen S, Rasmussen O, Ovesen J, Andersen K. Rotatory instability of cadaver knees after transaction of collateral ligaments and capsule. Arch Orthop Trauma Surg 1984;103:165–169
19. Nielsen S, Helmig P. Posterior instability of the knee joint: an experimental study. Arch Orthop Trauma Surg 1986;105:121–125

20. Grood ES, Stowers SF, Noyes FR. Limits of movement in the human knee: effect of sectioning the posterior cruciate ligament and posterolateral structures. J Bone Joint Surg 1988;70A:88–97
21. Cooper DE. Tests for posterolateral instability of the knee in normal subjects. J Bone Joint Surg 1991;73A:30–36
22. Veltri DM, Warren RF. Anatomy, biomechanics, and physical findings in posterolateral knee instability. Clin Sports Med 1994;13:599–614
23. Fanelli GC, Edson CJ. Posterior cruciate ligament injuries in trauma patients. Part II: arthroscopy 1995;11:526–529
24. Veltri DM, Deng X-H, Torzilli PA, Warren RF, Maynard MJ. The role of the cruciate and posterolateral ligaments in stability of the knee. Am J Sports Med 1995;23:436–443
25. Nielsen S, Helmig P. The static stabilizing function of the popliteal tendon in the knee: an experimental study. Arch Orthop Trauma Surg 1986;104:357–362
26. Kaneda Y, Moriya H, Takahaski K, Shimada Y, Tamaki T. Experimental study on external tibial rotation of the knee. Am J Sports Med 1997;25:796–800
27. Wroble RR, Grood ES, Cummings JS, Henderson JM, Noyes FR. The role of the lateral extraarticular restraints in the anterior cruciate ligament deficient knee. Am J Sports Med 1993;21:257–263
28. LaPrade RF, Konowalchuk BK. Popliteomeniscal fascicle tears causing symptomatic lateral compartment knee pain: diagnosis by the figure-4 test and treatment by open repair. Am J Sports Med 2005;33:1231–1236
29. Veltri DM, Deng X-H, Torzilli PA, Maynard MJ, Warren RF. The role of the popliteofibular ligament in stability of the human knee: a biomechanical study. Am J Sports Med 1996;24:19–27
30. Daniel DM, Stone ML, Barnett P, Sachs R. Use of the quadriceps active test to diagnose posterior cruciate ligament disruption and measure posterior laxity of the knee. J Bone Joint Surg 1988;70A:386–391
31. Stäubli HU. Posteromedial and posterolateral capsular injuries associated with posterior cruciate ligament insufficiency. Sports Med Arthro Rev 1994;2:146–164
32. Noyes FR, Barber-Westin SD. Surgical restoration to treat chronic deficiency of the posterolateral complex and cruciate ligaments of the knee joint. Am J Sports Med 1996;24:415–426
33. Noyes FR, Barber-Westin SD, Hewitt TE. High tibial osteotomy and ligament reconstruction for varus angulated anterior cruciate ligament deficient knees. Am J Sports Med 2000;28:282–296
34. Segond P. Recherches cliniques et experimentales sur les epanchcments snaguins du genou par entorse. Progress Med 1879;VII:1–84 (Paris)
35. Shindell R, Walsh WM, Connolly JF. Avulsion fracture of the fibula: the "arcuate sign" of posterolateral knee instability. Nebr Med J 1984;69:369–371
36. Kannus P. Nonoperative treatment of grade II and III sprains of the lateral ligament compartment of the knee. Am J Sports Med 1989;17:83–88
37. Woods GW, Stanley RF, Tullos HS. Lateral capsular sign: x-ray clue to a significant knee instability. Am J Sports Med 1979;7:27–33
38. LaPrade RF, Hamilton CD, Engebretsen L. Treatment of acute and chronic combined anterior cruciate ligament and posterolateral knee ligament injuries. Sports Med Arth Rev 1997;5:91–99
39. Johnson LL. Lateral capsular ligament complex: anatomical and surgical considerations. Am J Sports Med 1979;7:156–160

40. Terry GC, LaPrade RF. The biceps femoris muscle complex at the knee: its anatomy and injury patterns associated with acute anterolateral-anteromedial rotatory instability. Am J Sports Med 1996;24:2–8

41. DeLee JC, Riley MB, Rockwood CA. Acute posterolateral rotatory instability of the knee. Am J Sports Med 1983;11:199–207

42. Bousquet G, Charmion L, Passot JP, Girardin P, Relave M, Gazielly D. Stabilization du condyle externe du genou dans les laxiries anterieures chroniques. Rev Chir Orthop 1986;72:427–434

43. Noyes FR, Barber-Westin SD. Surgical reconstruction of severe chronic postero-lateral complex injuries of the knee using allograft tissues. Am J Sports Med 1995;23:2–12

44. Hassine D, Rougereau G, Feron JM, et al. MR imaging of posteromedial and pos-terolateral stabilizers of the knee: anatomic basis and patterns of lesions in knee injuries. Surg Radiol Anat 1994;16:293–301

45. Ruiz ME, Erickson SJ. Medial and lateral supporting structures of the knee, nor-mal MR imaging anatomy and pathologic findings. Magn Reson Imaging Clin N Am 1994;2:381–399

46. Seebacher JR, Inglis AE, Marshall JL, Warren RF. The structure of the posterolat-eral aspect of the knee. J Bone Joint Surg 1982;64A:536–541

47. Tardieu M, Lazennec JY, Christel P, Brasseur JL, Roger B, Grenier P. Normal and pathological MRI aspects of the posterolateral corner of the knee. J Radiol 1995;76:605–609

48. Brown TR, Quinn SF, Wensel JP, Kim JH, Demlow T. Diagnosis of popliteus in-juries with MR imaging. Skeletal Radiol 1995;24:511–514

49. Yu JS, Salonen DC, Hodler J, Haghighi P, Trudell D, Resnick D. Posterolateral as-pect of the knee: improved MR imaging with a coronal oblique technique. Radi-ology 1996;198:199–204

50. Ross G, Chapman AW, Newberg AR, Scheller AD Jr. Magnetic resonance imaging for the evaluation of acute posterolateral complex injuries of the knee. Am J Sports Med 1997;25:444–448

51. Miller MD, Gladden P, Staron RB, Henry JH, Feldman F. Posterolateral stabilizers of the knee: anatomy and injuries assessed with MR imaging. AJR Am J Roentgenol 1997;169:1641–1647

52. LaPrade RF, Gilbert TJ, Bollom TS, Wentorf F, Chaljub G. The magnetic resonance imaging appearance of individual structures of the posterolateral knee: a prospective study of normal knees and knees with surgically verified grade III injuries. Am J Sports Med 2000;28:191–199

53. LaPrade RF. Arthroscopic evaluation of the lateral compartment of knees with grade III posterolateral knee complex injuries. Am J Sports Med 1997;25: 596–602

54. Terry GC, LaPrade RF. The posterolateral aspect of the knee: anatomy and surgi-cal approach. Am J Sports Med 1996B;24:732–739

55. Stäubli HU, Birrer S. The popliteus tendon and its fascicles at the popliteus hia-tus: gross anatomy and functional arthroscopic evaluation with and without anterior cruciate ligament deficiency. Arthroscopy 1990;6:209–220

56. O'Brien SJ, Warren RF, Pavlov H, Panariello R, Wickiewicz TL. Reconstruction of the chronically insufficient anterior cruciate ligament with the central third of the patellar ligament. J Bone Joint Surg 1991;73A:278–286

57. Noyes FR, Barber-Westin SD. Revision of anterior cruciate surgery with use of bone-patellar tendon-bone autogenous grafts. J Bone Joint Surg 2001;83A:1131–1143

6

Clinically Relevant Biomechanics of Posterolateral Knee Injuries

Modern biomechanical testing of knee motion limits to determine the contribution of individual structures or groups of structures to knee stability has been performed since the mid-1970s,[1] when techniques were developed for continuous recordings of force and applied moments, displacement, and rotational relationships. Earlier biomechanical testing techniques had significant sources of potential error due to an inability to obtain precise measurements of the applied loads or motion achieved with an applied load. Those previous techniques included manual manipulation of the knees to apply loads, slings and weight-pulley systems to apply loads, and stress radiographs to measure motion.[2,3] Although these previous studies helped to improve the understanding of how structures contributed to knee instability, they lacked accuracy because many of the forces or applied moments to the knees were not known or controlled and the amount of displacement or rotation were either estimated or imprecisely measured as simultaneous displacement could not be recorded. For this reason, this chapter discusses only those biomechanical studies on the posterolateral knee that provide a quantitative measurement of the forces, moment displacements, or rotations tested.

Most biomechanical studies of the posterolateral knee have been studied largely through cadaveric sequential sectioning studies, in which the knee was subjected to joint loading before and after sectioning of a specific structure or group of structures. The resulting changes in joint motion were assessed and utilized to quantitate the contribution of the cut structure to overall knee stability for particularly applied loads. More recent studies have applied a given displacement to the joint, and measure the change in force present to create this displacement both before and after cutting individual specific posterolateral structures.

Many of the biomechanical studies about the posterolateral knee are difficult to compare with each other due to differences in nomenclature and the fact that many sequential cutting studies have grouped and sectioned these posterolateral structures together rather than studying them as individual structures. A review of the pertinent modern biomechanical studies of the posterolateral knee with an attempt to summarize which structures are important to primary and secondary knee stability follows. I have grouped the clinically relevant biomechanics into specific areas of motion testing to aid in the understanding of which structures may be injured for specific regions of instability abnormalities in patients with posterolateral knee injuries. The studies are summarized according to primary and secondary restraints. For those structures that are primary restraints, the instability being tested has found that structure which was cut or injured is the main restraint to that particular motion. Some structures provide secondary restraints to a particular motion when the primary restraint is absent. Also, it is important to recognize that injuries to the posterolateral corner of the knee are more complex than the lesions created in restraint and selective sectioning studies under static conditions in biomechanical testing laboratories.

◆ Role of the Posterolateral Structures in Preventing Varus/Valgus Motion

If one constant exists with respect to the stability provided to the posterolateral knee from a static biomechanical standpoint, it is that all studies have shown that the fibular collateral ligament is the primary restraint to varus motion in all positions of knee flexion.[1,4–9] Isolated sectioning of the fibular collateral ligament results in a significant increase in varus rotation at any knee flexion angle,[6–10] and varus rotation has not been demonstrated to be increased with posterolateral structure sectioning as long as the fibular collateral ligament is still intact.[6,9]

Grood et al[5] examined the restraints to varus opening of the knee at 5 and 25 degrees of knee flexion by measuring the forces necessary to create 5 mm of lateral joint line opening. They reported that at 5 degrees of knee flexion, the fibular collateral ligament was calculated to provide about 55% of the restraining moment to 5 mm of lateral joint line opening. The cruciate ligaments were calculated to contribute 22% to lateral restraint, the posterior capsule 13%, the iliotibial band and popliteus tendon 5%, and the anterior and midlateral capsule 4%. In comparison, at 25 degrees of knee flexion, the role of the fibular collateral ligament to restraining varus moment increased to 69%, whereas the role of the cruciates and combined capsule decreased to 12% and 9%, respectively. The role of the iliotibial band and popliteus tendon in providing lateral restraint was also slightly increased to 10%.

Many other structures have been found to be important in providing secondary varus stability to the knee when the fibular collateral ligament was sectioned. Nielsen et al[6] found a marked increase in varus opening of the knee with combined sectioning of the fibular collateral ligament and the posterolateral capsule of the knee, which was found to be maximal at 40 degrees of knee flexion. In another study, Nielsen et al[11] reported that combined posterior cruciate ligament (PCL), fibular collateral ligament, and posterolateral structure sectioning resulted in a marked increase in varus instability of the knee. Nielsen and Helmig[12] also found that the popliteus tendon had an important secondary role in preventing abnormal varus opening after the fibular collateral ligament was sectioned. They found that the maximal increase in varus opening again was at 40 degrees of knee flexion. Gollehon et al[8] sectioned the popliteus tendon and the posterolateral capsular structures, whereas Grood et al[9] cut the popliteus tendon attachment on the femur and the posterolateral part of the capsule, including the arcuate complex (which appears to be the popliteofibular ligament and capsular arm of the short head of the biceps femoris), along with the capsular attachment of the popliteus muscle (which appears to be the popliteal aponeurosis to the lateral meniscus) and any fabellofibular ligament or short lateral ligament that the authors found to be present after cutting the fibular collateral ligament. In both of these studies,[8,9] varus rotation was significantly increased with sectioning of these posterolateral knee structures compared with isolated fibular collateral ligament sectioning alone (**Figs. 6–1** and **6–2**). Veltri et al[10] found that additional sectioning

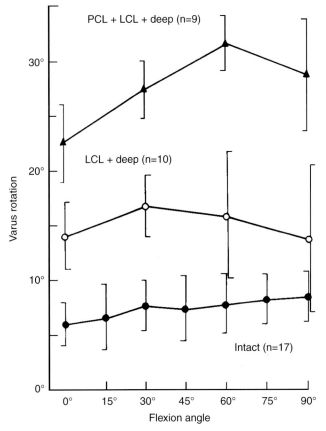

Figure 6–1   Varus opening with cutting posterolateral structures with 10 Newton-meters of varus torque applied. LCL, lateral collateral ligament; PCL, posterior cruciate ligament. (From Gollehon DL, Torzilli PA, Warren RF. The role of the posterolateral and cruciate ligaments in the stability of the human knee. A biomechanical study. J Bone Joint Surg 1987;69A:233–242, with permission.)

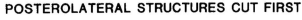

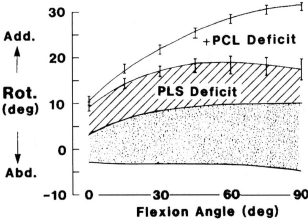

Figure 6–2   Varus opening with cutting posterolateral corner structures with application of a 20-newton meter torque. Shaded area, intact knees. Add., adduction (varus); abd., abduction (valgus); PLS, posterolateral structure. (From Grood ES, Stowers SF, Noyes FR. Limits of movement in the human knee. Effect of sectioning the posterior cruciate ligament and posterolateral structures. J Bone Joint Surg 1988;70A:88–97, with permission.)

of the popliteus tendon or popliteofibular ligament after the fibular collateral ligament was cut resulted in a significant further increase in varus rotation, which was found to be maximal at 30 degrees of knee flexion.

Studies have also shown that both cruciate ligaments are recruited to help resist an applied varus moment when the fibular collateral ligament and other posterolateral structures are absent. Gollehon et al[8] demonstrated that if the PCL was sectioned after the fibular collateral ligament and the deep posterolateral ligament complex were sectioned, a large increase in varus rotation occurred compared with isolated sectioning of the fibular collateral ligament at all knee flexion angles. Grood et al[9] also reported that cutting the PCL, after the fibular collateral ligament, popliteus tendon, and posterolateral structures were cut, resulted in increased varus rotation, which was maximally increased at 90 degrees. However, it has also been found that isolated PCL sectioning alone (with intact posterolateral knee structures) did not increase varus rotation of the knee.[8,9,11] Nielsen and Helmig[12] noted that the varus instability caused by anterior cruciate ligament (ACL) and fibular collateral ligament cutting could not be distinguished from isolated fibular collateral ligament cutting, and they postulated that the ACL could not be regarded as the primary varus stabilizer of the knee. Wroble et al[13] reported that isolated ACL sectioning resulted in no significant increase in varus opening at any knee flexion angle. They also demonstrated that in the ACL-deficient knee, cutting the fibular collateral ligament increased varus instability by only small amounts (at an average of 3 degrees), whereas additional sectioning of the posterolateral structures (which appear to be the popliteus and the associated posterolateral complex) produced larger secondary increases in varus opening at all knee flexion angles.

Markolf et al[14,15] reported that the resultant forces on the cruciate ligaments of cadaveric knees subjected to varus moments were significantly increased when the fibular collateral ligament and posterolateral structures were cut. They noted that when a varus moment was applied, the mean force on the native ACL was significantly increased when the posterolateral structures were cut compared with the intact state at all knee flexion angles. In addition, they reported that the native PCL, in a knee with intact posterolateral structures, was not loaded by varus moments applied to the knee. However, after the posterolateral structures were cut, the PCL became a main secondary restraint to an applied varus moment. When the posterolateral structures were cut, the PCL was found to have a significant increase in the mean force found on it at flexion angles greater than 45 degrees for an applied varus moment.[14] Maynard et al[16] performed mechanical strength testing of the fibular collateral ligament, popliteofibular ligament, and popliteus tendon (all three were pulled together) along the long axis of the fibular collateral ligament to simulate a pure varus injury to the knee. They found that tensile testing, at a rate of 100% per second, first resulted in failure of the fibular collateral ligament, at an average force to failure of 747 N, followed by failure of the popliteofibular ligament (with primarily intrasubstance tearing) at an average force to failure of 425 N, and failure of the popliteus tendon at its musculotendinous junction.

Therefore, in spite of many varying experimental models, the main structure that has been demonstrated to provide knee stability with application of a varus force is the fibular collateral ligament. In addition, the popliteus complex, posterolateral capsule, and cruciate ligaments have also been demonstrated to have an important secondary role in preventing varus instability when the fibular collateral ligament was cut. This means that if a knee does have an increase in varus opening on clinical examination, one must first suspect an injury to the fibular collateral ligament. Significant increases in a varus opening clinically would mean either a combined posterolateral structure injury or possibly a combined cruciate ligament tear is present.

Studies have not demonstrated any role of the posterolateral structures in preventing increased valgus motion.[6,8,13] Markolf et al[14] found that valgus angulation of the tibia was unaffected by sectioning of the fibular collateral ligament and posterolateral structures. In addition, they found no increase on force on either the anterior cruciate or PCL for an applied valgus moment with the posterolateral structures sectioned. Veltri et al[10] also found no greater than a 1-degree increase in primary valgus rotation of the knee for any isolated or combined posterolateral structure sectioning.

◆ Role of Posterolateral Structures in Preventing Anterior Translation

Selective sectioning studies have reported that cutting the posterolateral structures results in no significant increase in primary anterior tibial translation.[8,9,12] Veltri et al[10] found that for isolated posterolateral corner sectioning (which appears to include the fibular collateral ligament, popliteus tendon, popliteofibular ligament, and the capsular arm of the short head of the biceps femoris), there was no change in anterior translation of the knee with an anterior applied force at any knee flexion angle. Veltri et al[17] also found no significant change in anterior translation of the knee for posterolateral structure sectioning in a similar study. This would indicate that the posterolateral structures do not have a primary role in preventing anterior tibial translation of the knee. If one suspects an isolated posterolateral corner injury, there should not be any increase in anterior translation for the true Lachman test. However, there may be some increase in posterolateral motion, which may make it seem like there is an increased amount of relative anterior translation. In this instance, there should be a solid end point to the anterior Lachman test on clinical examination.

Nielsen and Helmig[12] found that anterior tibial displacement with the posterolateral capsule, popliteus tendon, and fibular collateral ligament sectioned was not increased until the ACL was also cut. They felt that this indicated that the posterolateral structures were an important secondary restraint to anterior tibial translation in the ACL-deficient knee. They also found that cutting the popliteus tendon or posterolateral structures in the ACL-deficient knee increased anterior tibial translation, most notably in the initial 40 degrees of knee flexion. They also noted that combined cutting of the ACL, popliteus tendon, and all posterolateral structures resulted in further increases in anterior translation instability up to 90 degrees of knee flexion.

Wroble[13] also found that in the ACL-deficient knee, cutting the fibular collateral ligament or posterolateral structures (the popliteus tendon and posterolateral capsule) produced small, but significant, increases in anterior tibial translation. They also reported that for combined sectioning of both the ACL and posterolateral structures, anterior tibial translation increased primarily near extension (in the initial 15 to 30 degrees of knee flexion), which they noted caused increased anterior translation that should be measurable clinically on the Lachman test.

In the ACL-deficient knee, the posterolateral structures that act as secondary restraints to anterior translation at 90 degrees of knee flexion have been found to include the iliotibial band, mid-third lateral capsular ligament, and the fibular collateral ligament.[18] In these ACL-deficient knees, the mean force contribution to anterior drawer at 90 degrees was calculated to be 25% for the iliotibial band, 21% for the mid-third lateral capsular ligament, and 12% for the fibular collateral ligament. The remaining forces were taken up by medial-sided structures.

Veltri et al[10] found results similar to those of other studies in knees in which the posterolateral structures were sectioned along with the ACL. In these knees, the authors found that significant increases in anterior translation occurred at all knee flexion angles for combined ACL and posterolateral structure sectioning compared with isolating sectioning of the posterolateral structures or for intact knees (**Fig. 6–3**). The maximal increase in anterior translation was found at 30 degrees of knee flexion for combined ACL and posterolateral structure sectioning. The authors stated that this indicated that the posterolateral structures were an important secondary stabilizer to anterior tibial translation.

A study that measured the force in the posterolateral knee structures, using a robotic/universal force-moment sensor testing system, revealed that the forces in the posterolateral structures were minimal with an intact ACL (<20 N), but that the forces present on the posterolateral structures when the ACL was sectioned increased by 123% at full knee extension and 413% at 15 degrees of knee flexion for an 134 N·m anteriorly applied force.[19] This would confirm the

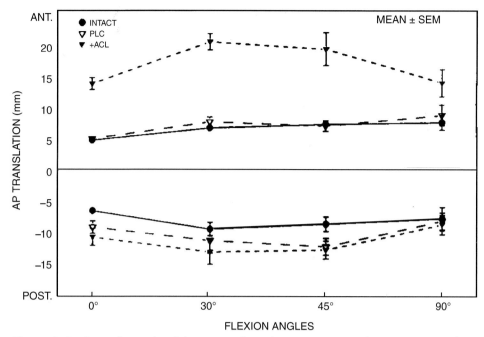

Figure 6–3 Secondary role of the posterolateral structures to preventing anterior tibial translation in the anterior cruciate ligament (ACL)-deficient knee resulting from a 100-newton meter anterior force, isolating sectioning if the posterolateral structures did not increase anterior translation at any flexion angle. PLC, posterolateral corner; ACL, anterior cruciate ligament. (From Veltri DM, Deng X-H, Torzilli PA, Warren RF, Maynard MJ. The role of the cruciate and posterolateral ligaments in stability of the knee. Am J Sports Med 1995;23: 436–443, with permission.)

results of other authors, who found that although the posterolateral knee structures play a minor role in resisting anterior tibial translation in an intact ACL knee,[8–10,12,17] they have a significant role in resisting anterior tibial translation in the ACL-deficient knee.[10,12,13] In analyzing Kanamori et al's[19] study, one could postulate that this information has very important implications for isolated repairs or reconstructions of torn posterolateral knee structures that occur in combination with an ACL tear. This study indicates that an isolated repair or reconstruction of torn posterolateral knee structures would be at risk for stretching out, if the ACL was not simultaneously reconstructed, because of the extra forces seen in the posterolateral structures with an ACL-deficient knee.

In summary, although the posterolateral structures do not have a primary role in preventing anterior tibial translation of the knee, they do play a very important role as a secondary restraint to anterior tibial translation in the ACL-deficient knee. In addition, the increase in anterior tibial translation seen with posterolateral corner injuries in a combined ACL tear should result in a significant increase in anterior tibial translation on the Lachman test that should be detectable clinically.[10,12,13] Therefore, in a knee with a 3+ or 4+ Lachman test and no other obvious ligament instability, including an intact posterior horn of the medial meniscus, the examiner must rule out a potential concurrent posterolateral knee injury. It has also been demonstrated that there is a significant increase in force on the posterolateral knee structures in an ACL-deficient knee. This important biomechanical finding supplements the clinical observation that, in combined posterolateral and cruciate ligament injuries, both the posterolateral structures and the cruciate ligament should be repaired or reconstructed concurrently at the original surgery, rather than during a staged surgery, to prevent the posterolateral structures from being stretched out.

◆ The Role of the Posterolateral Structures in Preventing Posterior Translation of the Tibia

It is very important to recognize that the main stabilizer of the knee with respect to primary posterior tibial translation is an intact PCL.[2,7,8,10,18,20] It is also important to recognize that the amount of posterior tibial translation that occurs with isolated sectioning of the PCL increases with increasing knee flexion angles. The greatest amount of measured posterior translation in the PCL-deficient knee was found to be at 90 degrees of knee flexion with values ranging from 1 to 5 mm at 0 degrees of knee flexion to 11 to 20 mm at 90 degrees of knee flexion.[8,9]

The posterolateral structures of the knee have been noted to play a significant primary, but minor, role in restricting posterior tibial translation. Gollehon et al[8] reported that isolated sectioning of the posterolateral structures resulted in at least a slight increase in posterior tibial translation at all angles of knee flexion. They also found that at 0 and 30 degrees of knee flexion there was no significant difference in posterior translation between specimens in which sectioning of the posterolateral structures was performed alone and those that have undergone isolated PCL sectioning **(Fig. 6–4)**. Grood et al[9] found that cutting all of the posterolateral structures resulted in a small, but significant, increase in posterior tibial translation from 0 to 45 degrees of knee flexion **(Fig. 6–5)**. In addition, Veltri et al[10] found that isolated sectioning of the posterolateral corner (which appears to have included the fibular collateral ligament, popliteus tendon, popliteofibular ligament, and the capsular arm of the short head of the biceps femoris) resulted in increases in posterior tibial translation with application of a posterior force at all angles of knee flexion with maximal increases occurring between 30 and 45 degrees of knee flexion. In a separate study, Veltri et al[17] also reported that isolated sectioning of the posterolateral structures affected primary posterior translation of the knee. Sectioning of the posterolateral structures increased posterior tibial translation at all degrees of knee flexion. Maximum primary posterior tibial translation was between 3.4 and 3.9 mm at between 30 and 45 degrees of knee flexion for isolated posterolateral structures sectioning. These studies[8–10,17] indicate that the posterolateral structures have a small but important primary role in preventing increased posterior tibial translation of the knee, especially near extension. This finding has important clinical significance in that the starting point of the tibia would be more posterior on the initial assessment of a Lachman's test with a posterolateral knee injury, which would be especially important with an intact ACL. The increase in anterior tibial translation from this "pseudo-Lachman" test may give the false impression of increased anterior tibial translation with an intact ACL. It is important to recognize that in these cases, the pseudo-Lachman test would have a solid end point, and the examiner in this case must carefully assess the integrity of the ACL.

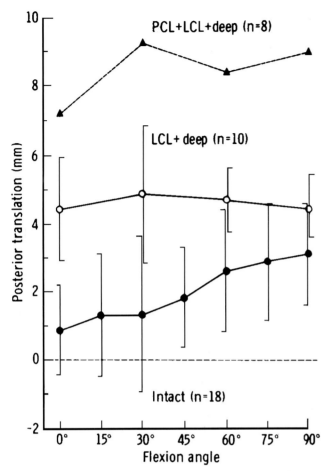

Figure 6–4 Increases in primary posterior translation with posterolateral knee structure cutting, compared with intact knees. Primary posterior translation increased more near the extension for lateral (fibular) collateral ligament (LCL) and deep structure sectioning, and posterior translation increased at 60° and 90° when the posterior collateral ligament (PCL) was also cut. (From Gollehon DL, Torzilli PA, Warren RF. The role of the posterolateral and cruciate ligaments in the stability of the human knee. A biomechanical study. J Bone Joint Surg 1987;69A:233–242, with permission.)

In addition to the minor primary role of the posterolateral knee structures in restricting posterior tibial translation, they have also been found to have an important secondary role in providing posterior stability in a PCL-deficient knee. Nielsen and Helmig[7] reported that combined cutting of the PCL, fibular collateral ligament, and posterolateral structures resulted in marked increases in posterior tibial translation, which became more important with increasing knee flexion. Gollehon et al[8] noted that combined PCL and posterolateral structures cutting resulted in a large increase in posterior tibial translation at all knee flexion angles. Grood et al[9] also reported that there was a significant further increase in posterior tibial translation after both the PCL and posterolateral structures were cut. Butler et al[18] found that the posterolateral capsule and popliteus tendon had a significant role in acting as a secondary restraint to posterior tibial translation when the PCL was cut at 90 degrees of knee flexion,

POSTEROLATERAL STRUCTURES CUT FIRST

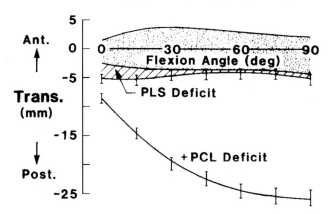

Figure 6–5   Increases in primary posterior tibial translation with posterolateral knee structure cutting. (From Grood ES, Stowers SF, Noyes FR. Limits of movement in the human knee. Effect of sectioning the posterior cruciate ligament and posterolateral structures. J Bone Joint Surg 1988;70A:88–97, with permission.)

whereas the iliotibial band and mid-third lateral capsular ligament had no primary or secondary role in resisting posterior tibial translation at 90 degrees. Although the medial collateral ligament complex, posteromedial capsule, mid-third medial capsular ligament, and fibular collateral ligament had some secondary role in preventing posterior tibial translation in a PCL-deficient knee, only the loss of the combined restraint of the posterolateral capsule and popliteus tendon was found to cause a significant increase in posterior tibial translation in a PCL-deficient knee.[18]

Nielsen and Helmig[7] found that in the PCL-deficient knee, the popliteus tendon was the structure that had the largest effect on resisting posterior tibial translation from 10 to 90 degrees of knee flexion when it was cut **(Fig. 6–6)**. Others have also demonstrated that combined sectioning of the PCL and posterolateral structures of the knee significantly increased posterior tibial translation compared with isolating sectioning of either the PCL or the posterolateral structures individually.[8,9]

Markolf et al[14] measured the force in the PCL with a posteriorly applied 50-N force with concurrent fibular collateral ligament and posterolateral corner structure sectioning. They found that the mean force on the PCL was unaffected by sectioning of these posterolateral structures for a straight posteriorly applied force.

Harner et al[21] evaluated the effect of a simulated contraction of the popliteus muscle on both the forces seen on the native PCL and in knee kinematic changes for a 110-N posteriorly applied load (which simulated a posterior drawer test) using a cadaveric robotic model. They found that a simulated 44-N contraction of the popliteus muscle resulted in significantly decreased in situ forces seen on the native PCL at both 30 and 90 degrees of knee flexion. In addition, they found that after cutting the PCL, the amount of posterior translation of the tibia was reduced by up to 36% with a simulated popliteus muscle contraction. They concluded that this demonstrated the popliteus muscle dynamically resists posterior tibial translation with the PCL, and an intact and

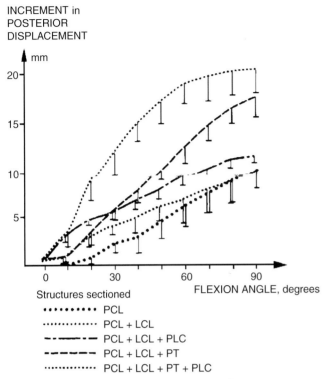

INCREMENT in
POSTERIOR
DISPLACEMENT

Structures sectioned

•••••••• PCL

•••••••••••• PCL + LCL

–•–––•– PCL + LCL + PLC

––––– PCL + LCL + PT

•••••••••••• PCL + LCL + PT + PLC

Figure 6–6   The role of the popliteus tendon on increases in posterior knee translation during sequential structure sectioning and a 25-newton meter positively directed force. PCL, posterior increase ligament; LCL, lateral (fibular) collateral ligament; PLC, posterolateral corner; PT, popliters tendon. (From Nielsen S, Helmig P. The static stabilizing function of the popliteal tendon in the knee: an experimental study. Arch Orthop Trauma Surg 1986;104:357–362, with permission.)

functional popliteus complex can help with improved knee stability in the PCL-deficient knee. They confirmed the clinical observation by Barnett and Richardson[22] that the popliteus complex provides active support to the PCL in resisting posterior subluxation of the tibia on the femur in the flexed knee.

In summary, the posterolateral structures of the knee act as a minor, but significant, primary restraint to posterior tibial translation across all angles of knee flexion,[8–10,17] but the PCL is the main primary stabilizer for these posterior translation movements.[2,7,8,10,18,20] The role of primary restraint of the posterolateral structures of the knee to posterior tibial translation is most important between 0 and 30 degrees of knee flexion, where the amount of posterior tibial translation may be as much as for a knee with an isolated posterolateral corner injury as for an isolated PCL tear.[8,9] This has clinical importance in a knee with a posterolateral corner injury in that these may be a false impression of anterior translation on the Lachman test or pseudo-Lachman test in a knee with an intact ACL. In a PCL-deficient knee, the posterolateral structures also act as an important secondary stabilizer to posterior translation of the knee. When the posterolateral structures and the PCL were both cut, a significant further increase in posterior translation was seen compared with isolated cutting of either structure.[7–9,18] This has important clinical significance because most

2+ posterior drawer tears have an isolated PCL tear, whereas most 3+ posterior drawer tests knee combined PCL and posterolateral structure injuries. This information has been found to be important in the assessment of increased posterior translation on PCL stress radiographs. As mentioned previously, most isolated PCL tears have less than 1 cm of increased posterior translation on PCL stress x-rays. However, increases on posterior translation equal to or greater than 12 mm are almost always an indication of a combined PCL and posterolateral corner injury (or a possible combined posteromedial knee injury).

◆ Role of the Posterolateral Structures in Preventing Internal Rotation at the Knee

Lipke et al[23] measured motion changes with ACL and anterolateral/posterolateral structure cutting between 0 and 40 degrees of knee flexion. They reported that isolated fibular collateral ligament and posterolateral complex (described as the lateral capsule and ligament structures) sectioning resulted in no significant increase in internal rotation until the ACL was also cut. They also found a significant increase in internal rotation when the ACL was cut, and further additional internal rotation occurred with cutting the fibular collateral ligament or posterolateral structures. They did not assess higher knee flexion angles in their biomechanical testing studies.

However, other studies performed at varying knee flexion angles have shown that when an internal rotation torque was placed on the knee, an isolated or combined loss of the fibular collateral ligament, deep or posterolateral structures (the popliteus complex and posterior joint capsule), or PCL caused a significant increase in primary internal rotation of the tibia.[6,9,24] In addition, Veltri et al[10] found a small, but significant, increase in internal tibial rotation with the posterolateral structures cut compared with intact knees. However, the maximal increase was only 2.9 degrees at 90 degrees of knee flexion. The small increase in primary internal rotation seen in other studies may explain why it was not found in Lipke et al's[23] study.

Nielsen et al[6] reported that cutting the fibular collateral ligament and the posterolateral knee structures resulted in increased internal rotation at flexion angles greater than 50 degrees. Nielsen et al[11] also noted no increase in primary internal tibial rotation with isolated PCL sectioning. In addition, Wroble et al[13] demonstrated that in the ACL-deficient knee, the posterolateral structures (which appear to be the popliteus complex and posterolateral capsule in their study) had an important role as a secondary stabilizer in preventing internal tibial rotation, which was most important close to knee extension.

Markolf et al[14] measured the forces generated in the cruciate ligaments when the posterolateral structures were cut and found the mean force on the ACL increased at 0, 10, and 20 degrees of knee flexion, but not at higher knee flexion angles, for an applied internal rotation torque. They found no change in PCL force at any knee flexion angle with the posterolateral structures sectioned for any applied internal rotation torque.[14]

In summary, it appears that the posterolateral structures play a small role in preventing primary internal rotation of the knee. In addition, they play an important role as a secondary restraint to internal rotation in the ACL-deficient knee, especially when the knee is close to extension. However, due to the varied amount of internal rotation changes and the large standard deviations seen for this test, this particular knee instability has not been shown to have much clinical significance to date in motion testing. Perhaps further study into its clinical significance and the development of a clinical test to measure this motion abnormality may be indicated.

◆ Role of the Posterolateral Structures in Preventing External Rotation at the Knee

The integrity of the posterolateral structures has been demonstrated to be very important in preventing increased primary external rotation of the knee. Lipke et al[23] found that with cutting all the structures of the posterolateral complex, a significant increase in external rotation was found between 0 and 40 degrees of knee flexion. However, they did not assess this affect at higher knee flexion angles. Nielsen et al[6] found no change in external rotation of the knee with isolated fibular collateral ligament cutting and minimal changes with isolated posterolateral structures (everything except the fibular collateral ligament) sectioning. They found a large increase in external rotation, however, with an average of 15.6 degrees, at 30 degrees of knee flexion and a 10.2-degree increase in external rotation at 70 degrees of knee flexion, with combined fibular collateral ligament and posterolateral capsule sectioning. They found the maximal increase in external rotation was at 35 degrees of knee flexion. Nielsen et al[11] noted a significant increase in external rotation occurred with combined PCL, fibular collateral ligament, and posterolateral structure sectioning, which increased with increasing knee flexion. They postulated that this would indicate that the PCL is an important secondary stabilizer to external rotation at knee flexion angles greater than 35 degrees. Nielsen and Helmig[12] found a significant increase in external rotation for isolated popliteus tendon sectioning between 20 and 130 degrees of knee flexion. They found the largest increased amount of external rotation (16 degrees) occurred at 30 degrees of knee flexion with the fibular collateral ligament, popliteus tendon, and posterolateral corner structures cut. Further flexion of the knee under these same cutting conditions resulted in a decrease in the amount of external rotation with ~7 degrees of increased external rotation compared with an intact knee occurring at 90 degrees of knee flexion.

Gollehon et al[8] also demonstrated the importance of intact posterolateral structures with respect to external tibial rotation. They noted that isolated sectioning of the fibular collateral ligament, as well as the popliteus complex, resulted in a significant increase in external tibial rotation at all knee flexion angles compared with intact knees (**Fig. 6–7**). Grood et al[9] found that after sectioning of the posterolateral structures (which appear to have been the fibular collateral ligament, popliteofibular ligament, fabellofibular ligament, capsular arm of the short head of the biceps femoris, and the popliteus tendon femoral attachment), a significant increase in external tibial rotation occurred at both 30 and

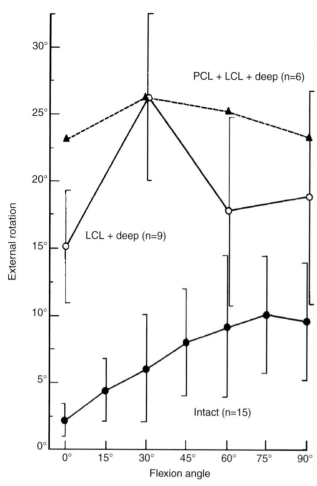

Figure 6–7   Couples increases in external rotation with isolated posterolateral knee structure cutting and a 100 W posteriorly applied force. PCL, posterior cruciate ligament; LCL, lateral (fibular) collateral ligament. (From Gollehon DL, Torzilli PA, Warren RF. The role of the posterolateral and cruciate ligaments in the stability of the human knee. A biomechanical study. J Bone Joint Surg 1987;69A:233–242, with permission.)

90 degrees of knee flexion (13 and 5.3 degrees of increase, respectively) **(Fig. 6–8)**. Veltri et al[10] also found that cutting the fibular collateral ligament, popliteus tendon, and popliteofibular ligament resulted in an increase in external rotation at all angles of knee flexion, which was maximum at 45 degrees. In addition, Kaneda et al[25] verified some of these previous studies,[8,9] using biplanar roentgenographic photogrammetry and assessed the effect of cutting the posterolateral structures on external tibial rotation of the knee. They found that sectioning the fibular collateral ligament and the posterolateral structures (which appear to have been the popliteofibular ligament, fabellofibular ligament, popliteus tendon, and the capsular arm of the short head of the biceps femoris) resulted in significant increases in external tibial rotation at 30, 60, and 90 degrees of knee flexion compared with the intact knee state. The clinical significance of these biomechanical studies is that the dial test at 30 and 90 degrees for examination of the knee is based on the results found in these biomechanical studies.[7–10,25]

POSTEROLATERAL STRUCTURES CUT FIRST

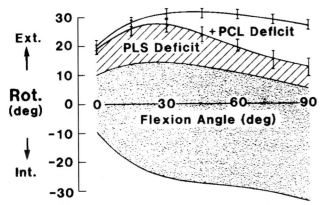

Figure 6–8 Increases in external rotation with isolated posterolateral knee structure (PLS) cutting versus combined posterior cruciate ligament (PCL) and posterolateral structure (PLS) sectioning. Shaded area, intact knee. (From Grood ES, Stowers SF, Noyes FR. Limits of movement in the human knee. Effect of sectioning the posterior cruciate ligament and posterolateral structures. J Bone Joint Surg 1988;70A:88–97, with permission.)

Markolf et al[14] found that the force measured on the native ACL when the posterolateral structures were cut decreased at 0, 10, and 20 degrees when an external rotation torque was applied. Wroble et al[13] found that the posterolateral structures restrained external rotation at all knee flexion angles and that isolated ACL cutting resulted in a clinically insignificant increase in external rotation of the knee (<1 degree). They also found that in the ACL-deficient knee, an intact fibular collateral ligament limited any increase in external rotation to less than 4 degrees for any knee flexion angle (between 0 and 90 degrees) with the posterolateral structures (popliteus and posterolateral capsule) sectioned. The fibular collateral ligament was noted to limit external rotation at all knee flexion angles, with the most important effect near extension. Further cutting of the fibular collateral ligament at this point resulted in an increase of external rotation, compared with the intact state, of greater than 14 degrees at all knee flexion angles compared with the posterolateral structures intact state. In addition, Wroble et al[13] found that in the ACL-deficient knee with the fibular collateral ligament and posterolateral structures sectioned, a significant increase in external rotation compared with the intact state was seen at all knee flexion angles with a maximal increase in external rotation occurring at 90 degrees of knee flexion (which was 15 degrees). However, Veltri et al[10] found that in the ACL-deficient knees of their study, the increase in primary external rotation measured with cutting the fibular collateral ligament, popliteus tendon, and popliteofibular ligament did not differ from that found in intact knees. They suggested that the dial test to assess for posterolateral instability may not be clinically reliable at 30 degrees because it may not pick up combined ACL and posterolateral knee injuries, and they implied that this finding might explain why posterolateral injuries that occur with a concurrent ACL tear are often missed. This study appears to have findings in contrast to the study of Wroble et al[13] for the amount of external rotation seen at both 30 and 90 degrees for a combined ACL–posterolateral knee injury.

In a separate study, Nielsen et al[11] found that isolated PCL cutting resulted in no significant increase in external rotation of the knee with an applied external rotation torque. Nielsen and Helmig[7] also found that a marked increase in external rotation occurred, which increased from 0 to 40 degrees, with a maximum at 23 degrees of knee flexion, with combined PCL, fibular collateral ligament, and posterolateral structure sectioning that remained fairly constant with increasing knee flexion. Gollehon et al[8] found that when the PCL was cut after the posterolateral structures, a significant increase in external rotation was seen at 60 and 90 degrees of knee flexion compared with isolated posterolateral corner sectioning. Grood et al[9] also found that isolated PCL sectioning did not increase external rotation at any knee flexion angle. However, when the PCL was sectioned after the posterolateral structures, an additional increase in external rotation was also noted, but this was significant only at 90 degrees of knee flexion. Kaneda et al[25] also found that isolated PCL sectioning alone did not increase the amount of external tibial rotation. However, cutting the PCL after the fibular collateral ligament and posterolateral structures were cut resulted in a significant increase in external tibial rotation at 60 and 90 degrees of knee flexion. They reported that this indicated that the PCL acts as an important secondary restraint to external rotation in a knee with a posterolateral corner injury at higher knee flexion angles. In addition, Markolf et al[14] found that the mean force generated in the PCL with an external rotation torque applied, with the posterolateral structures sectioned, increased at flexion angles greater than 45 degrees.

In summarizing the role of the posterolateral structures in preventing external tibial rotation, the fibular collateral ligament, popliteus tendon, and popliteofibular ligament have been found to be the primary stabilizers to external rotation of knees with the largest increase in external rotation seen at 30 degrees of knee flexion (13 to 16 degrees) when these structures were cut.[6,7,9,12] In addition, both the PCL[8,9,25] and the ACL[13] have been found to be important secondary stabilizers to external tibial rotation of the knee in biomechanical testing performed at 90 degrees of knee flexion, which should be detectable clinically as increased external rotation of the knee on the dial test at 90 degrees. Normally, for an isolated posterolateral knee injury, there should be a decrease in external rotation when the dial test is performed at 90 degrees compared with 30 degrees of knee flexion. In addition, isolated ACL or PCL injury should not result in increased external tibia rotation at any knee flexion angle.[8,11,13] This has clinical importance in that any increase of external rotation on the dial test at 30 or 90 degrees in an ACL or PCL injury would indicate the likelihood of a concurrent posterolateral corner knee injury.

◆ Role of Posterolateral Structures in Preventing Coupled Anterior Translation, Internal Rotation and Posterior Translation, and External Rotation Motion

When an anterior force is applied in the normal intact knee, the tibia tends to rotate internally.[8,13,20] When an anterior force is applied to the knee with the posterolateral structures, PCL, or fibular collateral ligament sectioned, there is a small but significant further increase in coupled internal tibial rotation.[10,23] Nielsen and Helmig[12] also noted that combined sectioning of the ACL, fibular collateral ligament, and the posterolateral structures, leaving the popliteus tendon intact, resulted in a small increase in internal rotation. A marked increase in coupled external rotation was seen when the popliteus tendon was also cut, which was noted to be a maximum of 15 degrees at 70 degrees of knee flexion.

A posteriorly applied force to the normal knee results in coupled external rotation of the tibia.[8,20,26] In a knee with an intact posterolateral corner, an applied coupled posterior drawer and external rotation torque results in no significant increase in force on either the ACL or the PCL.[14] Nielsen and Helmig[12] noted a significant increase in coupled external rotation with posterolateral structure cutting only from 20 to 60 degrees of knee flexion, whereas others have found that combined sectioning of the fibular collateral ligament and popliteus tendon caused a marked increase in coupled external rotation associated with a posterior directed force at all angles of knee flexion.[10,14,24] Nielsen and Helmig[7] also noted that combined sectioning of the PCL, fibular collateral ligament, and posterolateral structures resulted in an increased amount of coupled external rotation with a posteriorly applied force to the knee.

Jakob et al[27] sectioned the mid-third lateral capsular ligament, fibular collateral ligament, and popliteus tendon in various sequences and combinations to help determine the pathomechanics necessary to produce a reverse pivot shift test in cadaveric knees. They found that the popliteus tendon and its expansion to the lateral meniscus (the popliteal aponeurosis to the lateral meniscus) was the main structure that prevented the reverse pivot shift. Sectioning the fibular collateral ligament resulted in a slight amount of laxity for the reverse pivot shift test. Sectioning the mid-third lateral capsular ligament and lateral gastrocnemius did not contribute any instability to the reverse pivot shift test. Nielsen and Helmig[7] were also able to reproduce a reverse pivot shift when an anterior force was applied to the knee with the PCL and all the posterolateral structures sectioned when the knee was flexed at about 30 to 40 degrees of knee flexion. They also reported that the popliteus tendon played a major role in preventing this posterolateral subluxation.

Markolf et al[14] found that the mean force on the native PCL for a combined 50-N posterior force and a coupled 7-N·m external rotation torque was significantly increased at all knee flexion angles, except at full extension, for the posterolateral structures cut state compared with the intact state. They reported that the increase in force was significantly greater for combined posterior drawer–external rotation loads than for an external rotation torque alone.

Although it is clear that a posterolateral knee complex injury will result in a significant increase in coupled posterior translation and external rotation of the knee, the role of the PCL in providing coupled external rotation is less clear. Jakob et al[27] found a significant increase of combined posterior translation and external rotation with sectioning of both the PCL and the posterolateral structures. Gollehon et al[8] suggested that an isolated loss of the PCL equated to a complete loss of coupled external rotation when a posterior force was applied and that there was also a nonsignificant increase of coupled external rotation with a posterior force with combined PCL and posterolateral structure cutting. In addition, Veltri et al[10] found that sectioning the PCL after the posterolateral structures were cut resulted in an increase in coupled external rotation only at 0 degrees of knee flexion.

The clinical significance of these findings is in the assessment of coupled posterolateral rotation of the knee. The main coupled motion that is detected clinically is for the combined posterior drawer and external rotation movement seen clinically for both the reverse pivot shift and posterolateral drawer tests.

Popliteomeniscal Fascicles and Lateral Meniscal Stability

Simonian et al[28] evaluated the stability of the lateral meniscus both before and after cutting the anteroinferior and posterosuperior popliteomeniscal fascicles. They found that with application of a 10-N anterior load to the lateral meniscus, the average lateral meniscal anterior motion in the intact state was 3.6 mm. With the popliteomeniscal fascicles sectioned, the average anterior motion of the lateral meniscus with a 10-N load was significantly increased to 6.4 mm. They found that the anteroinferior popliteomeniscal fascicle was larger and provided greater stability to the lateral meniscus than the thinner posterosuperior popliteomeniscal fascicle. They noted that the lateral meniscus did not become anteriorly locked in any of the knees in the study with the 10-N load applied, and it spontaneously reduced to its original position once it was unloaded. They theorized that with the loads seen during normal daily activities, mechanical symptoms might be expected when the popliteomeniscal fascicles were torn and meniscal motion was significantly increased. Their studies confirm the clinical observation of Stäubli and Birrer,[29] who reported that the popliteomeniscal fascicles became tensioned with a varus moment applied to the knee and prevented medial displacement of the lateral meniscus into the joint.

◆ Effects of a Posterolateral Knee Injury on Joint Line Contact Force at the Knee

Skyhar et al[30] studied the effects of sectioning the PCL and the popliteus muscle and tendon, fibular collateral ligament, and the posterolateral capsule on alterations of contact pressure within the knee in 10 cadaveric knees using Fuji pressure/sensitive film. In addition to finding a significant increase in contact pressures in the patellofemoral joint and the medial compartment with cutting the PCL, the highest elevation of the contact pressures in these joints was seen with additional combined sectioning of the posterolateral knee structures. The authors concluded that patients with combined PCL and posterolateral knee injuries need to be informed about the increased risk of osteoarthritis of these compartments if these injuries were not treated. In addition, Skyhar et al found a significant increase in quadriceps load at 15 and 90 degrees of knee flexion for combined sectioning of the PCL and posterolateral knee structures compared with isolated PCL sectioning. They felt that this was due to increased posterior tibial subluxation and the resultant increase in stress on the quadriceps muscle group after combined sectioning of these structures.

The clinical importance is that these biomechanical studies support the clinical observations of Kannus[31] that patients with posterolateral corner injuries have a higher incidence of osteoarthritis over time. It is especially important to counsel patients with combined PCL and posterolateral knee injuries that they are at a high risk for the development of osteoarthritis if their ligament injuries are not treated.

Fibular Collateral Ligament Elongation During Motion Testing of the Posterolateral Knee

It has been postulated that the biceps femoris complex can exert a compressive force on the fibular collateral ligament, thus exerting a stabilizing force on the lateral side of the knee. We performed a study to compare the difference in elongation of the fibular collateral ligament in response to loaded and unloaded conditions on the biceps femoris muscle-tendon complex during clinical motion testing for the posterolateral knee.

Six fresh-frozen cadaveric lower extremities were minimally dissected to identify the fibular collateral ligament with preservation of the lateral aponeurotic attachments from the long and short heads of the biceps femoris to the fibular collateral ligament. A differential variable reluctance transducer (DVRT) (Microstrain, Burlington, VT) was implanted into the midsubstance of the fibular collateral ligament at its slack-taut transition to measure the local strain of the ligament. The specimen was mounted into a specially designed frame with the femoral shaft fixed intramedullarly and the following muscle-tendon units were loaded by a pulley system: quadriceps (44 N); medial hamstrings (gracilis, semimembranosus, semitendinosus) (22.5 N); medial and lateral gastrocnemius (22.5 N); and the iliotibial band (10 N). The load on the biceps complex varied depending on the experimental condition (22.5 N, loaded; 2 N, unloaded). Motion testing was then performed for both the loaded and unloaded states for the following tests: Lachman test, posterolateral tibial rotation at 30 degrees (posterolateral Lachman test), varus at 0 degrees, varus at 30 degrees, posterolateral drawer, and the dial tests at 30 and 90 degrees. Each clinical test was performed three times and the repeatability of the clinical testing was verified.

The average percent elongation (local strain) of the fibular collateral ligament was as follows: Lachman test (6.2%, loaded; 4.9%, unloaded), posterolateral tibial rotation at 30 degrees of flexion (8.3%, loaded; 7.1%, unloaded), varus at 0 degrees (9.5%, loaded; 7.9%, unloaded), varus at 30 degrees (13.3%, loaded; 13.4%, unloaded), posterolateral drawer (8.0%, loaded; 7.9%, unloaded), dial test at 30 degrees (9.4%, loaded; 4.9%, unloaded), and the dial test at 90 degrees (10.2%, loaded; 8.0%, unloaded). There were no significant differences in percent elongation of the fibular collateral ligament for clinical motion testing of the posterolateral knee in the biceps femoris loaded versus unloaded state.

We were unable to prove a possible dynamic role of the biceps in providing strain relief to the fibular collateral ligament through its lateral aponeurotic attachments during clinical limits-of-motion tests specific for the posterolateral knee. It is possible that dynamic stability may be granted through a more complex mechanism through the multiple attachments of the biceps femoris complex to the posterolateral knee that we were unable to detect. The clinical tests that produced the most local strain of the fibular collateral ligament were varus at 30 degrees of knee flexion, the dial test at 90 degrees, and varus at 0 degrees of knee flexion.

The Measurement of Elongation of Specific Posterolateral Knee Structures During Clinical Motion Testing

Our aims in this project were to measure the elongation of specific posterolateral knee structures to clinical loads specific for the posterolateral knees. Measurements were performed for a loaded knee, both before and after sequential cutting of structures, to determine which structures exhibited the greatest local strain for specific clinical tests and how these values varied with cutting of the posterolateral structures of the knee.

Six fresh-frozen cadaveric lower extremities were dissected to isolate the mid-third lateral capsular ligament, fibular collateral ligament, popliteofibular ligament, oblique popliteal ligament, ligament of Wrisberg, and the anterolateral bundle of the PCL. The anteromedial bundle of the ACL was identified through a small medial parapatellar incision. Anatomic relationships between structures were preserved whenever possible. DVRT strain transducers were implanted into the midsubstance of the structures at the slack-taut transition of the structure to measure the percent elongation (local strain) of the structures. The specimen was then mounted into a specially designed frame with the femoral shaft fixed intramedullarly and the following muscle-tendon units loaded to a pulley system: quadriceps (44 N); medial hamstrings (gracilis, semimembranosus, semitendinosus) (22.5 N); biceps femoris (22.5 N); medial and lateral gastrocnemius (22.5 N); and the iliotibial band (10 N). Motion testing was then performed utilizing the following tests: Lachman test, varus at 30 degrees, posterolateral tibial rotation at 30 degrees (posterolateral Lachman test), posterolateral drawer, and the dial test at 30 and 90 degrees. After testing in the normal state, sequential cutting studies of the popliteofibular ligament, fibular collateral ligament, the mid-third lateral capsular ligament, and the popliteus origin on the femur were performed with replication of the clinical motion tests.

The greatest percent elongations (local strains) of posterolateral knee structures for specific clinical motion testing were as follows: Lachman test (mid-third lateral capsular ligament, 15.4%; fibular collateral ligament, 6.0%), varus at 30 degrees (mid-third lateral capsular ligament, 14.1%; popliteofibular ligament, 13.1%; fibular collateral ligament, 13.1%); posterolateral tibial rotation at 30 degrees (popliteofibular ligament, 18.3%; mid-third lateral capsular ligament, 16.2%; fibular collateral ligament, 8.4%), posterolateral drawer (popliteofibular ligament, 25.0%; mid-third lateral capsular ligament, 10.6%; fibular collateral ligament, 9.1%), dial test at 30 degrees (popliteofibular ligament, 20.3%; mid-third lateral capsular ligament, 12.7%; fibular collateral ligament, 10.0%), and the dial test at 90 degrees (popliteofibular ligament, 30.5%; fibular collateral ligament, 12.1%; mid-third lateral capsular ligament, 12.1%). The ligament of Wrisberg and oblique popliteal ligament exhibited very little (<4%) elongation across all posterolateral clinical testing in the intact knees.

Statistically significant increases in local strain were seen for the following structures during sequential cutting studies: Lachman test—popliteofibular ligament cut; fibular collateral ligament ($p < .04$) and oblique popliteal ligament ($p < .05$); posterolateral tibial rotation at 30 degrees—popliteofibular ligament cut; fibular collateral ligament ($p < .04$); and the dial test at 30 degrees—popliteofibular ligament cut; mid-third lateral capsular ligament ($p < .03$). No significant increase in percent elongation was seen for the cruciate ligaments.

In this study, preservation of the major anatomic structures (and their complex interattachments), along with loading the knee, allowed for a more complete analysis of the interrelationships of the complex anatomy of the posterolateral knee. Posterolateral tibial rotation at 30 degrees (posterolateral Lachman test) and the dial test at 30 degrees of knee flexion demonstrated differential increases in the amounts of strain of the secondary restraints with sequential cutting studies of the posterolateral knee. It appears that both tests are useful to assess the integrity of the secondary restraints of the posterolateral knee. The ligament of Wrisberg and the oblique popliteal ligament were found to have little local strain through all posterolateral clinical motion testing and appear to have little primary role in preventing posterolateral rotatory instability of the knee.

Direct Force Measurements of the Posterolateral Knee Structures to Applied Loads

Although the selective sectioning method of assessing the importance of a specific structure, or group of posterolateral knee structures, does provide useful information about the structure and the static stability of the knee, sectioning the structures changes the intricate interactions and relationships of the remaining posterolateral knee structures. This means that the results obtained from selective sectioning depends on the sequence in which the structures are cut. Therefore, the conclusions about the contribution of a specific posterolateral knee structure to overall knee stability are obtained indirectly rather than on direct measurements.

Although most of our knowledge about the relative importance of individual anatomic structures of the posterolateral knee in providing static knee stability is derived from sequential cutting studies, there has been a paucity of studies that directly measure the forces on these structures during joint loading. It is important to determine these direct forces to allow us to assess whether reconstructive procedures for posterolateral corner injuries reproduce the same relative loading of these native structures in the uninjured state. Thus, it is important to recognize that the measurement of the relative direct force on structures during joint loading is necessary to determine if surgical reconstructive procedures can replicate the relative function of the structures that they replace.

Quantitative measurement of ligament strain on force includes the use of Hall effect transducers,[32] liquid-filled strain gauges,[33] and buckle transducers.[34,35] Ligament strain measurements are usually expressed as relative to the measurement of the ligament length for a particular knee flexion angle and load application.

Direct measurements of forces seen in the fibular collateral ligament, popliteus tendon, and popliteofibular ligament to applied loads have been taken by the use of buckle transducers.[36] The buckle transducer consists of a stainless steel frame with a semiconductor strain gauge mounted on a removable crossbar. The crossbar of the buckle transducer is inserted under the ligament and then pulled through the frame held on top of the ligament

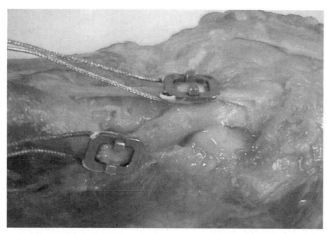

Figure 6–9 A popliteofibular ligament and fibular collateral ligament with buckle transducers in place for measurement of force seen on the structure to applied loads.

(Fig. 6–9). Loads applied to the knee cause crossbar deflection if the particular structure is loaded. The amount of the crossbar deflections is quantified by strain gauges attached to the crossbar. The strain gauges are connected to a Wheatstone bridge, which connects to a data acquisition system that quantifies the forces.

In our study, custom-made buckle transducers were placed around the fibular collateral ligament, popliteus tendon, and popliteofibular ligament. High relative loads were seen on the fibular collateral ligament for both varus and external rotation. The highest amount of force seen on the fibular collateral ligament was at 0 degrees of knee flexion with external rotation, with the mean load response decreasing with higher knee flexion amounts **(Fig. 6–10)**. Fibular collateral ligament varus load response at 0, 30, and 60 degrees was found to be fairly constant with a significance decrease at 90 degrees compared with 30 degrees of knee flexion **(Fig. 6–11)**. The load response of the fibular collateral ligament to internal rotation was variable and demonstrated no significant differences among 0, 30, 60, or 90 degrees of knee flexion. In this study, the popliteus tendon and popliteofibular ligament were loaded with an external rotation moment and had similar loading patterns **(Fig. 6–10)**. The mean popliteus tendon and popliteofibular ligament load response peaked at 60 degrees of knee flexion. We found that there was a reciprocal relationship of load sharing in external rotation, depending on the knee flexion angle, which had not been recognized previously with the selective cutting studies. We found that the force present on the fibular collateral ligament with external rotation loads was much higher than the popliteus complex at lower flexion angles, whereas the popliteus complex had higher load sharing than the fibular collateral ligament at 60 and 90 degrees of knee flexion. In this regard, we found that the fibular collateral ligament was more highly loaded with an external rotation torque in the early ranges of knee motion (0 to 30 degrees) and to be significantly more loaded than the popliteus complex. From this information, we concluded that the fibular collateral ligament has a very important role in preventing external rotation at early knee flexion that had not been emphasized or recognized in previous posterolateral knee cutting studies.

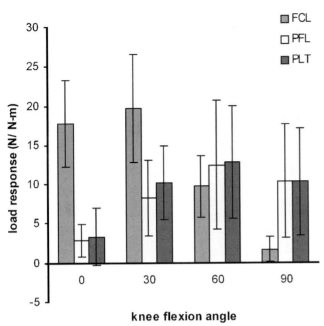

Figure 6–10   Fibular collateral ligament (FCL), popliteus tendon (PLT), and popliteofibular ligament (PFL) load response to an external rotation torque of 6 N·m. (From LaPrade RF, Tso A, Wentorf FA. Force measurements on the fibular collateral ligament, popliteofibular ligament, and popliteus tendon to applied loads. Am J Sports Med 2004;32:1695–1701, with permission.)

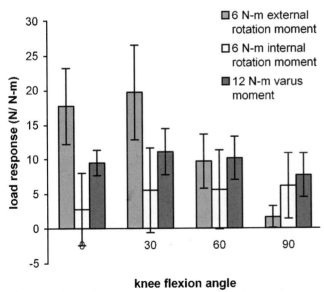

Figure 6–11   Fibular collateral ligament load response to varus and internal/external rotation stress testing. (From LaPrade RF, Tso A, Wentorf FA. Force measurements on the fibular collateral ligament, popliteofibular ligament, and popliteus tendon to applied loads. Am J Sports Med 2004;32:1695–1701, with permission.)

Although it was found that the fibular collateral ligament was highly loaded with an external rotation torque in lower knee flexion angles, the popliteus tendon and popliteofibular ligament were more highly loaded with higher degrees of knee flexion. From this information, it appears that the fibular collateral ligament and the popliteus complex, which includes the popliteus tendon and the popliteofibular ligament, have complementary roles as external rotation stabilizers of the knee that had not been appreciated previously. The fibular collateral ligament has a much more important role in preventing external rotation near extension, whereas the popliteus complex assumes a more important primary role in preventing external rotation with increasing knee flexion.

It has been well recognized in previous selective sectioning studies of the posterolateral knee that knees do not have a significant increase in varus opening unless the fibular collateral ligament is sectioned. Our direct force measurements also found this to be significantly true. We found that the varus moments on the knee caused a high amount of force to be seen on the fibular collateral ligament at all knee flexion angles that were tested, whereas the popliteus tendon and the popliteofibular ligament did not have any significant increase in force generated on them with these knee flexion angles with the fibular collateral ligament intact. In addition, it was also found that application of an anterior, posterior, or valgus applied force did not load the fibular collateral ligament, popliteus tendon, or popliteofibular ligament.

It is important to recognize that little has been known in the past about the forces seen on the main structures of the posterolateral knee with applied loads. To properly plan a reconstructive procedure, it is important to determine which structures should be reconstructed and the relative strengths needed for the reconstructive grafts. The information that is gained from measurement of the direct forces reveals that the fibular collateral ligament not only has an important role in preventing varus opening of the knee but also has an important primary role in preventing external rotation of the knee near extension that has not been well recognized. In addition, the direct force measurement technique also verified that the popliteus complex has an important primary role in preventing external rotation of the knee at higher knee flexion angles. Therefore, it is possible that some of the difficulties in obtaining good outcomes in fibular collateral ligament reconstruction procedures, which often have been found to have a high amount of residual laxity, may be due to a lack of understanding of this role.

◆ Effects of Tensioning of Cruciate Ligament Grafts and the Integrity of the Posterolateral Knee Structures on Tibiofemoral Orientation

Wentorf et al[37] assessed the effects of tensioning an ACL graft and the integrity of the posterolateral knee structures on tibiofemoral orientation. We found a significant increase in tibial external rotation occurred with increasing ACL graft tension in the presence of a posterolateral knee injury compared with the posterolateral structures intact state (**Fig. 6–12**). We recommended repairing or reconstructing the posterolateral knee injuries first, prior to ACL graft fixation

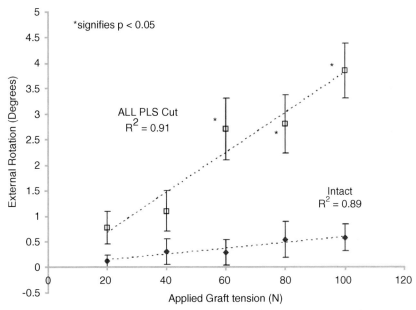

Figure 6–12   Amount of tibiofemoral external rotation seen with anterior cruciate ligament graft tightening with posterolateral structures (PLS) cut. (From Wentorf FA, LaPrade RF, Lewis JL, Resig S. The influence of the integrity of posterolateral structures on tibiofemoral orientation when an anterior cruciate ligament graft is tensioned. Am J Sports Med 2002;30:796–799, with permission.)

on the tibia (with the ACL graft already secured in the femoral tunnel), to reduce the risk of an external rotation deformity of the knee with combined ACL and posterolateral knee injuries. We did not assess the effect of holding the extremity (foot) in neutral rotation when securing the ACL graft in the tibial tunnel. It is possible that holding the tibia in neutral while securing the ACL graft in the tibial may prevent the external rotation deformity from occurring.

In addition, we assessed the effects of tensioning a PCL graft and the integrity of the posterolateral knee structures on tibiofemoral orientation (unpublished data, 1999). We found no difference in tibiofemoral orientation with either the posterolateral structures intact or sectioned when the PCL graft was tensioned at 90 degrees of knee flexion. Therefore, we recommend that the PCL graft be secured first to provide a restoration of the central pivot to the knee, in the face of a combined PCL reconstruction and a concurrent posterolateral corner repair or reconstruction, and that the posterolateral structures be repaired or tensioned after the PCL graft is secured.

◆ Effect of a Proximal Tibial Opening Wedge Osteotomy on Posterolateral Knee Instability

We have performed biomechanical testing of the results of a proximal tibial opening wedge osteotomy on the change in stability of knees with posterolateral corner knee injuries. This study was performed because of the clinical observation that there was increased stability in knees that underwent a proximal tibial opening wedge osteotomy for the treatment of chronic posterolateral corner knee injuries. Biomechanical testing was performed on cadaveric knees in the intact state, after transection of the fibular collateral ligament, popliteus tendon, and popliteofibular ligament, and after a 10-mm proximal tibial opening wedge osteotomy.

We found that after transection of the posterolateral corner structures, varus opening increased by a mean of 6 mm to varus stressing at both 30 and 90 degrees of knee flexion. After performing a proximal tibial opening wedge osteotomy, varus opening decreased by a mean of 3 mm at both 30 and 90 degrees of knee flexion. External rotation of the knee was found to increase after posterolateral knee structure sectioning by 5 degrees at 30 degrees of knee flexion and 6 degrees at 90 degrees of knee flexion after posterolateral structure sectioning compared with the intact state. After the proximal tibial opening wedge osteotomy was performed, external rotation significantly decreased back to baseline at 30 degrees of knee flexion and was overconstrained by 1 degree at 90 degrees of knee flexion compared with the intact state.

Our results demonstrated that a 10-mm proximal tibial opening wedge osteotomy decreased varus translation and external rotation motion for knees that had a posterolateral knee deficiency. A buckle transducer that was placed on the tibial collateral ligament found that there was increased force observed in the tibial collateral ligament, especially with respect to varus and external rotation applied loads, which may help explain the increased stability pattern observed in posterolateral corner knee injuries after a proximal tibial opening wedge osteotomy.

The clinical importance of this study is that it confirmed that a proximal tibial opening wedge osteotomy can tighten up the soft tissues around the knee in the face of a posterolateral corner knee injury with a secondary decrease in varus translation and external rotation instability. This may explain clinically why some patients have good function and do not need a second-stage soft tissue reconstruction of their posterolateral knee structures after undergoing a proximal tibial opening wedge osteotomy for the treatment of a combined genu varus and a grade 3 posterolateral corner knee injury.

◆ Effects of Posterolateral Knee Injuries in Forces Seen on Cruciate Ligament Reconstructions

In one of our studies, we tried to determine if untreated injuries of the posterolateral structures of the knee contribute to increased force on an ACL reconstruction graft (which could potentially lead to graft failure) compared with the intact posterolateral knee state.[38] We used the selective ligament cutting technique to determine the effects of sectioning specific posterolateral knee structures on the forces seen on an ACL reconstruction graft to applied loads compared with its baseline state (with intact posterolateral knee structures) for specific applied forces.

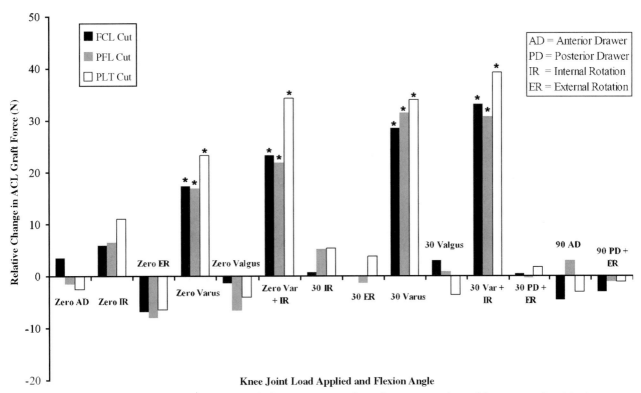

Figure 6–13 Anterior cruciate ligament graft forces seen with posterolateral knee structure cutting to applied forces. (From LaPrade RF, Resig S, Wentorf FA, Lewis JL. The effects of grade III posterolateral knee complex injuries on anterior cruciate ligament graft force. A biomechanical analysis *= PL.05. Am J Sports Med 1999;27:469–475, with permission.)

Anterior cruciate ligament graft force was significantly higher after cutting the fibular collateral ligament during varus loading at both 0 degrees and 30 degrees of knee flexion than it was for the same loading at the joint with intact posterolateral knee structures (**Fig. 6–13**). In addition, coupled loading of varus and internal rotation moments at 0 and 30 degrees of knee flexion further increased graft force beyond that found with varus moments alone. The increase in graft force remained significant with additional sequential cutting of the popliteofibular ligament and popliteus tendon. Because an internal rotation moment by itself did not result in a significant increase in ACL graft force, we theorized that the main abnormal motion that increased the load seen on the ACL graft when there was a concurrent posterolateral knee injury was a varus moment.

Extrapolation of the loads applied in our study to the study by Prodromos et al[39] of adduction moments during gait yields some rough comparisons of the force on an ACL graft in vivo in a knee with a posterolateral injury with uncorrected varus instability. Prodromos et al found some patients in their study had an adduction moment of 6% of their body weight (BW) × height (HT). In comparing the highest average increase in graft force seen in this study, 71 N (for coupled varus and internal rotation at 0 degrees of flexion), to a proportional increase to the joint varus moment seen in Prodromos et al's study, their values need to be converted to Newton-meters. With a typical mean male body weight of 155 pounds (690 N) and height of 1.8 m, 6% × BW × HT becomes 75 Nm. Converting this adduction moment of 75 Nm proportionally to the 12-Nm applied load (torque) in our study [75 Nm/12 Nm × 71 N (the highest load)], would theoretically result in 444 N of increased force on the ACL graft under these conditions. Rowden et al[40] reported that the failure strength of a patellar tendon ACL graft averages 416 N immediately after reconstruction. In addition, because animal studies have shown that ACL grafts weaken with time before gaining strength after remodeling after an ACL reconstruction,[41-43] the forces that may occur on an ACL graft for a patient with an untreated posterolateral knee injury and a varus thrust gait could cause the graft to rupture or stretch out in the initial period after surgical reconstruction.

Therefore, we strongly recommend that either a repair or reconstruction of torn posterolateral structures, especially in knees with evidence of varus instability, be performed at the time of ACL reconstruction to reduce the risk of ACL graft failure. In addition, due to the fact that a tightened ACL graft (fixed in both tunnels) may initially overconstrain the knee and mask the amount of abnormal motion from a posterolateral knee injury, it is recommended that a decision to repair or reconstruct a posterolateral corner injury be made prior to ACL graft fixation. This would need to be based on an examination under anesthesia, and possibly supplemented with an arthroscopic evaluation of the lateral compartment, if it had not been previously diagnosed by the clinical examination or MRI evaluation. If this is not done, then a pathologic amount of posterolateral joint laxity may not be recognized, due to the fixed ACL graft overconstraining the knee with a posterolateral knee injury, which could lead to failure of the ACL reconstruction graft with time and activity.

Harner et al[44] also evaluated the effect of deficient posterolateral knee structures on a PCL reconstruction using a robotic/universal force-moment sensor testing system. In an isolated PCL injury model, a PCL reconstruction restored posterior tibial translation to within 1.5 mm of the normal intact knee at 30 degrees and 2.4 mm at 90 degrees of knee flexion with a 134-N posterior tibial load applied to the knee. In the same testing conditions with the posterolateral knee structures cut (the fibular collateral ligament and popliteus complex), posterior tibial translation was 6.0 mm at 30 degrees and 4.6 mm at 90 degrees compared with the intact knee. In addition, external rotation increased by up to 14 degrees whereas varus rotation increased up to 7 degrees for the cut compared with the intact posterolateral knee structures state. Calculated in situ forces in the PCL graft were noted to significantly increase for a 134-N posterior tibial load (at 30 and 90 degrees), a 5-N·m external rotation torque, a coupled 67-N posterior drawer/2.5-N·m external rotation torque, and 5-N·m varus torque loading conditions for the posterolateral structures cut state. The authors concluded that PCL grafts are rendered ineffective and may be overloaded in the presence of posterolateral knee structure deficiency. They recommended that both the PCL and posterolateral structures be reconstructed concurrently in a combined knee ligament injury.

We also tried to determine if untreated posterolateral knee injuries contribute to a significant increase in force on a PCL reconstruction graft compared with the posterolateral structures' intact state (which could potentially lead to graft failure).[45] Joint loading was performed on the knees after a PCL reconstruction with the posterolateral structures intact, followed by sequential individual sectioning and testing of the popliteofibular ligament, popliteus tendon, and fibular collateral ligament with concurrent measurements recorded of the load changes on the PCL graft.

A significant increase in force was seen on the PCL reconstruction graft when the popliteofibular ligament, popliteus tendon, and fibular collateral ligament were cut compared with the posterolateral structures intact state with application of both a varus moment and a coupled posterior drawer and external rotation torque (**Fig. 6–14**) at 30, 60, and 90 degrees of knee flexion. Clinical motion testing should be able to detect these motion abnormalities through the varus stress test at 30 degrees, the dial test at 30 and 90 degrees, the posterolateral drawer test, and the reverse pivot shift test.[5,8–10,13,27,46–49] It is believed that the findings of this study verify the clinical observation that a failure to repair or reconstruct posterolateral knee injuries at the time of PCL reconstruction

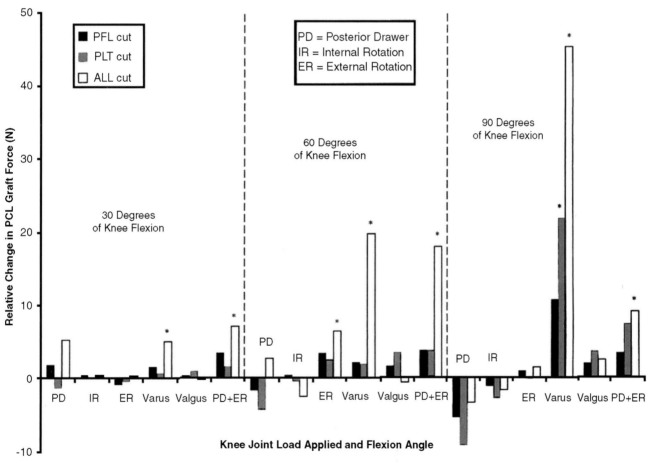

Figure 6–14 Posterior cruciate ligament graft forces seen with posterolateral knee structure cutting to applied forces [* = statistically significant changes ($p <.05$)]. (From LaPrade RF, Muench CW, Wentorf FA, Lewis JL. The effect of injury to the posterolateral structures of the knee on force in a posterior cruciate ligament graft. A biomechanical study. * = PL.05. Am J Sports Med 2002;30:233–23, with permission.)

places the PCL reconstruction graft at risk for failure by significantly increasing the force placed on it.

It is recommended that knees with PCL tears and combined posterolateral knee injuries, especially those with evidence of varus and/or coupled posterior drawer/external rotation instability, have concurrent posterolateral knee repair or reconstruction at the time of PCL reconstruction to reduce the risk of PCL graft failure. In addition, due to the PCL graft potentially overconstraining the knee immediately after graft fixation when the posterolateral structures are deficient and masking the amount of abnormal joint motion from the posterolateral knee injury, it is recommended that a decision to repair or reconstruct the posterolateral knee injury be made prior to PCL graft fixation (either on the exam under anesthesia or with a concurrent arthroscopic evaluation of the lateral compartment if it had not been diagnosed previously via the physical examination or MRI evaluation). Otherwise, the overconstrained PCL graft would potentially limit the amount of abnormal knee motion due to the posterolateral knee injury, which could result in a failure to recognize the severity of the posterolateral knee injury, if one were relying on an exam under anesthesia after PCL graft fixation. This failure would lead to extra force on the PCL graft, which could lead to PCL reconstruction graft failure.

Mechanical Failure Properties of the Posterolateral Structures of the Knee

It is important to understand the structural properties of the main static stabilizers of the posterolateral knee (fibular collateral ligament, popliteus tendon, and popliteofibular ligament) to assist with the selection of reconstructive graft choices for anatomic posterolateral knee reconstructive techniques. Three studies have been performed that have attempted to look at these properties.

Maynard et al[50] simultaneously stretched the fibular collateral ligament and popliteofibular ligament to failure along the long axis of the fibular collateral ligament. The mean tensile strengths of the fibular collateral ligament and popliteofibular ligament using this testing technique were 750 N and 425 N, respectively. However, because these structures were not individually tested, the data obtained cannot be viewed as representative of the strength of the individual ligaments.

Two other studies have looked at the individual strengths of these posterolateral knee structures. Sugita and Amis[51] found that the individual tensile strengths of the fibular collateral ligament and popliteofibular ligament were 309 N and 180 N, respectively. However, these authors did not individually test the strengths of the popliteus tendon.

We have also performed testing on the mechanical failure properties of the posterolateral structures of the knee.[52] In this study, each structure was individually isolated and loaded to failure at a rate greater than 100% per second. We found the average mean ultimate tensile strength of the fibular collateral ligament was 295 N, the popliteofibular ligament was 229 N, and the popliteus tendon was 680 N. The average cross-sectional areas of these same structures at their midpoints were 11.9 mm^2, 17.1 mm^2, and 21.9 mm^2, respectively. The clinical significance of this information is that we found that the popliteofibular ligament, fibular collateral ligament, and popliteus tendon can resist fairly large loads prior to failure. We recommend that the average graft strength chosen for posterolateral knee reconstructions meet or exceed these findings.

Biomechanical Analysis of an Anatomic Posterolateral Knee Reconstruction

Based on our quantitative anatomy studies of the posterolateral corner of the knee for the attachment sites of the fibular collateral ligament, popliteus tendon, and popliteofibular ligament,[53] we developed an anatomic surgical technique to reconstruct these structures[54] (see Chapter 7). Utilizing the University of Minnesota knee joint testing system, we found that this surgical reconstructive technique significantly improved varus joint stability at 0, 30, 60, and 90 degrees of knee flexion. In addition, significant improvement was found in external rotation between the reconstructive and the cut state. We found that this anatomic posterolateral knee reconstructive technique, using two separate grafts to reconstruct the fibular collateral ligament, popliteus tendon, and popliteofibular ligament, restored static varus and external rotation stability in cadaveric knees. In addition, there was no biomechanical evidence of this reconstructive technique overconstraining the knees, which has been found to occur with the biceps tenodesis procedure.[55] It was felt that the anatomic placement of the grafts would allow for early unrestricted knee motion, which has been borne out through further clinical studies. In addition, this reconstructive technique does not rely on the use of local dynamic or static stabilizing structures, which could result in morbidity in those posterolateral reconstructive techniques that utilize them.[55–58] The details of this anatomic posterolateral corner reconstructive procedure are presented in Chapter 7.

◆ Assessment of Healing of Posterolateral Knee Injuries

We performed an in vivo sectioning study of the fibular collateral ligament and popliteus tendon in a group of 14 New Zealand white rabbits. At 3 months postoperatively, only one rabbit had healed the sectioning, with the remaining knees demonstrating a significant increase in lateral joint opening to an applied varus stress. This study confirmed the clinical observations of Kannus,[31] who found that grade 3 posterolateral knee injuries usually did not heal and that patients had generally poor function if they were not treated.[59]

◆ Summary of the Literature Review on the Biomechanics of the Posterolateral Knee

In spite of the differences in nomenclature, the order in which posterolateral knee structures have been sectioned, the varying experimental protocols in sequential static biomechanical cutting studies, and the differences between the apparent roles of these structures in providing static stability to the posterolateral knee, the findings are fairly consistent. Overall, the main structures of the posterolateral knee found to prevent abnormal motion are the fibular collateral ligament, popliteus tendon, and popliteofibular ligament.[1,4–10,12,17]

The primary role that the posterolateral structures play in restraint is in preventing abnormal varus and external rotation motion.[5–10,12,17] The posterolateral structures of the knee also play a small role in primary posterior translation, especially in the first 30 degrees of knee flexion,[8,9,17] and in primary internal rotation motion of the knee.[6,9,10,24]

In addition, the posterolateral structures have been found to be important secondary stabilizers to posterior translation of the knee from 0 degrees to 90 degrees of flexion and to anterior translation when the knee is near extension.[7–10,12,13,17] The posterolateral structures have also been found to be important secondary stabilizers in internal rotation in the ACL-deficient knee, especially between 0 and 30 degrees of flexion.[13,14]

The fibular collateral ligament is the main structure that provides stability to varus moments of the knee.[1,4–6,8,9,12] The components of the popliteus complex and posterolateral capsule also play an important role in preventing secondary varus instability.[6–10,12]

Both the fibular collateral ligament and the popliteus complex (consisting of the popliteus tendon and popliteofibular ligament) have been found to have an important role in providing stability against an external rotation force to the knee.[6,8–10,12,36] Significant increases in external tibial rotation have been found with cutting these structures. It has not been clearly defined which structure is most important in preventing an increase in external rotation with posterolateral knee injuries, but it appears that the fibular collateral ligament may be more important in the initial stages of knee flexion, and the popliteus tendon and popliteofibular ligament have more importance in increasing amounts of knee flexion in preventing external rotation instability.[36]

There does not appear to be a clear role for which structures contribute to prevention of posterior translation with sectioning of posterolateral knee structures, especially in the initial phases of knee flexion. The popliteus tendon has some role in this regard, especially with higher knee flexion angles, but the role of the other posterolateral knee structures is less well defined.[12]

In summary, the main structures that have been identified through selective cutting studies to prevent increases in the joint motion seen with static biomechanical testing of the posterolateral knee are the fibular collateral ligament, popliteus tendon, and popliteofibular ligament. The role of other posterolateral knee structures in preventing this increase in abnormal motion is less clear, as individually cutting these other posterolateral knee structures has not been performed. In addition, the biomechanical role of the integrity of the posterolateral knee structures on the forces on either an ACL or PCL has been defined only recently. In light of the recognition of the role of deficient posterolateral knee structures on cruciate ligament graft failures clinically,[60–62] combined with biomechanical studies that demonstrate that deficiencies of these posterolateral structures place a significant increase in force on both ACL and PCL reconstructive grafts, it is highly recommended that the posterolateral structures be repaired or reconstructed at the time of cruciate ligament reconstruction to prevent increases in forces on these reconstructions that could lead to graft failure. In addition, it is especially important to make the decision to perform a repair or reconstruction of the posterolateral structures at the time of the examination under anesthesia or during the diagnostic arthroscopy,[49] and not after fixation of the cruciate ligament reconstruction grafts. It has been demonstrated that the cruciate ligament grafts will overconstrain the knee[21,38,45] in the face of cruciate ligament graft fixation and mask the underlying instability of the knee caused by a posterolateral knee injury. In addition, as previously mentioned, failure to repair or reconstruct the posterolateral structures in this instance would place a high amount of increased stress on the cruciate ligament graft, which would place them at high risk for failure.

References

1. Markolf KL, Mensch JS, Amstutz H. Stiffness and laxity of the knee—the contributions of the supporting structures. J Bone Joint Surg 1976;58A:583–594
2. Brantigan OC, Voshell AF. The mechanics of the ligaments and menisci of the knee joint. J Bone Joint Surg 1941;23A:44–66
3. Ouellet R, Levesque HP, Laurin CA. The ligamentous stability of the knee: an experimental investigation. Can Med Assoc J 1969;100:45–50
4. Seering WP, Piziali RL, Nagel DA, Schurman DJ. The function of the primary ligaments of the knee in varus-valgus and axial rotation. J Biomech 1980;13: 785–794
5. Grood ES, Noyes FR, Butler DL, Suntay WJ. Ligamentous and capsular restraints preventing straight medial and lateral laxity in intact human cadaver knees. J Bone Joint Surg 1981;63A:1257–1269
6. Nielsen S, Rasmussen O, Ovesen J, Andersen K. Rotatory instability of cadaver knees after transaction of collateral ligaments and capsule. Arch Orthop Trauma Surg 1984;103:165–169
7. Nielsen S, Helmig P. Posterior instability of the knee joint: an experimental study. Arch Orthop Trauma Surg 1986;105:121–125
8. Gollehon DL, Torzilli PA, Warren RF. The role of the posterolateral and cruciate ligaments in the stability of the human knee: a biomechanical study. J Bone Joint Surg 1987;69A:233–242
9. Grood ES, Stowers SF, Noyes FR. Limits of movement in the human knee: effect of sectioning the posterior cruciate ligament and posterolateral structures. J Bone Joint Surg 1988;70A:88–97
10. Veltri DM, Deng X-H, Torzilli PA, Warren RF, Maynard MJ. The role of the cruciate and posterolateral ligaments in stability of the knee. Am J Sports Med 1995;23:436–443
11. Nielsen S, Ovesen J, Rasmussen O. The posterior cruciate ligament and rotatory knee stability: an experimental study. Arch Orthop Trauma Surg 1985;104: 53–56
12. Nielsen S, Helmig P. The static stabilizing function of the popliteal tendon in the knee: an experimental study. Arch Orthop Trauma Surg 1986;104:357–362
13. Wroble RR, Grood ES, Cummings JS, Henderson JM, Noyes FR. The role of the lateral extraarticular restraints in the anterior cruciate ligament deficient knee. Am J Sports Med 1993;21:257–263
14. Markolf KL, Wascher DC, Finerman GA. Direct *in vitro* measurement of forces in the cruciate ligaments. Part II: the effects of section of the posterolateral structures. J Bone Joint Surg 1993;75A:387–394

15. Markolf KL, Burchfield DM, Shapiro MM, Cha CW, Finerman GA, Slauterbeck JL. Biomechanical consequences of replacement of the anterior cruciate ligament with a patellar ligament allograft. Part II: forces in the graft compared with forces in the intact ligament. J Bone Joint Surg 1996;78A:1728–1734

16. Maynard MJ, Deng X-H, Wickiewicz TL, Warren RF. The popliteofibular ligament: rediscovery of a key element in posterolateral instability. Am J Sports Med 1996;24:311–316

17. Veltri DM, Deng X-H, Torzilli PA, Maynard MJ, Warren RF. The role of the popliteofibular ligament in stability of the human knee: a biomechanical study. Am J Sports Med 1996;24:19–27

18. Butler DL, Noyes FR, Grood ES. Ligamentous restraints to anterior-posterior drawer in the human knee. J Bone Joint Surg 1980;62A:259–270

19. Kanamori A, Sakane M, Zeminski J, Rudy TW, Woo SW. In-situ force in the medial and lateral structures of intact and ACL-deficient knees. J Orthop Sci 2000;5:567–571

20. Fukubayashi T, Torzilli PA, Sherman MF, Warren RF. An in vitro biomechanical evaluation of anterior-posterior motion of the knee: tibial displacement, rotation, and torque. J Bone Joint Surg 1982;64A:258–264

21. Harner CD, Höher J, Vogrin TM, Carlin GJ, Woo SL-Y. The effects of a popliteus muscle load on in situ forces in the posterior cruciate ligament and on knee kinematics. Am J Sports Med 1998;26:669–673

22. Barnett CH, Richardson AT. The postural function of the popliteus muscle. Ann Phys Med 1953;1:177–179

23. Lipke JM, Janecki CJ, Nelson CL, et al. The role of incompetence of the anterior cruciate and lateral ligaments in anterolateral and anteromedial instability. J Bone Joint Surg 1981;63A:954–960

24. Noyes FR, Stowers SF, Grood ES, Cummings J, VanGinkel LA. Posterior subluxations of the medial and lateral tibiofemoral compartments: an in vitro ligament sectioning study in cadaveric knees. Am J Sports Med 1993;21:407–414

25. Kaneda Y, Moriya H, Takahaski K, Shimada Y, Tamaki T. Experimental study on external tibial rotation of the knee: a m J Sports Med 1997;25:796–800

26. Torzilli PA, Greenberg RL, Insall J. An in vivo biomechanical evaluation of anterior-posterior motion of the knee. J Bone Joint Surg. 1981;63A:960–968

27. Jakob RP, Hassler H, Stäubli HU. Observations on rotatory instability of the lateral compartment of the knee: experimental studies on the functional anatomy and pathomechanism of the true and reversed pivot shift sign. Acta Orthop Scand Suppl 1981;191:1–32

28. Simonian PT, Sussman PS, van Trommel M, Wickiewicz TL, Warren RF. Popliteomeniscal fasciculi and lateral meniscal stability. Am J Sports Med 1997;25:849–853

29. Stäubli HU, Birrer S. The popliteus tendon and its fascicles at the popliteus hiatus: gross anatomy and functional arthroscopic evaluation with and without anterior cruciate ligament deficiency. Arthroscopy 1990;6:209–220

30. Skyhar MJ, Warren RF, Ortiz GJ, Schwartz E, Otis JC. The effects of sectioning of the posterior cruciate ligament and the posterolateral complex on the articular contact pressures within the knee. J Bone Joint Surg 1993;75A:694–699

31. Kannus P. Nonoperative treatment of grade II and III sprains of the lateral ligament compartment of the knee. Am J Sports Med 1989;17:83–88

32. Arms S, Pope MH, Johnson RJ, Fischer RA, Arvidsson I, Eriksson E. The biomechanics of anterior cruciate ligament rehabilitation and reconstruction. Am J Sports Med 1984;12:8–17

33. Monahan JJ, Grigg P, Pappas AM, et al. *In vivo* strain patterns in the four major canine knee ligaments. J Orthop Res 1984;2:408–418

34. Ahmed AM, Hyder A, Burke DL, Chan KH. *In vitro* ligament tension pattern in the flexed knee in passive loading. J Orthop Res 1987;5:217–230

35. Lewis JL, Lew WD, Hill JA, et al. Knee joint motion and ligament forces before and after ACL reconstruction. J Biomech Eng 1989;111:97–106

36. LaPrade RF, Tso A, Wentorf FA. Force measurements on the fibular collateral ligament, popliteofibular ligament, and popliteus tendon to applied loads. Am J Sports Med 2004;32:1695–1701

37. Wentorf FA, LaPrade RF, Lewis JL, Resig S. The influence of the integrity of posterolateral structures on tibiofemoral orientation when an anterior cruciate ligament graft is tensioned. Am J Sports Med 2002;30:796–799

38. LaPrade RF, Resig S, Wentorf FA, Lewis JL. The effects of grade III posterolateral knee complex injuries on anterior cruciate ligament graft force: a biomechanical analysis. Am J Sports Med 1999;27:469–475

39. Prodromos CC, Andriacchi TP, Galante JO. A relationship between gait and clinical changes following high tibial osteotomy. J Bone Joint Surg 1985;67A: 1188–1194

40. Rowden NJ, Sher D, Rogers GJ, Schindhelm K. Anterior cruciate ligament graft fixation: initial comparison of patellar tendon and semitendinosus autografts in young fresh cadavers. Am J Sports Med 1997;25:472–478

41. Butler DL, Grood ES, Noyes FR, et al. Mechanical properties of primate vascularized vs. nonvascularized patellar tendon grafts: changes over time. J Orthop Res 1989;7:68–79

42. Jackson DW, Grood ES, Goldstein JD, et al. A comparison of patellar tendon autograft and allograft used for anterior cruciate ligament reconstruction in the goat model. Am J Sports Med 1993;21:176–185

43. Ng GY, Oakes BW, Deacon OW, McLean ID, Lampard D. Biomechanics of patellar tendon autograft for reconstruction of the anterior cruciate ligament in the goat: three-year study. J Orthop Res 1995;13:602–608

44. Harner CD, Vogrin TM, Höher J, Ma BC, Woo SL-Y. Biomechanical analysis of a posterior cruciate ligament reconstruction: deficiency of the posterolateral structures as a cause of graft failure. Am J Sports Med 2000;28:32–39

45. LaPrade RF, Muench CW, Wentorf FA, Lewis JL. The effect of injury to the posterolateral structures of the knee on force in a posterior cruciate ligament graft: a biomechanical study. Am J Sports Med 2002;30:233–238

46. Hughston JC. Knee ligament injuries in athletes. Med J Alabama 1966;36: 243–252

47. Hughston JC, Andrews JR, Cross MJ, Moschi A. Classification of knee ligament injuries. Part I: the medial compartment and cruciate ligaments. J Bone Joint Surg 1976;58A:159–172

48. Hughston JC, Norwood LA. The posterolateral drawer test and external rotation recurvation test for posterolateral rotatory instability of the knee. Clin Orthop Rel Res 1980;147:82–87

49. LaPrade RF, Terry GC. Injuries to the posterolateral aspect of the knee: association of anatomic injury patterns with clinical instability. Am J Sports Med 1997;25:433–438

50. Maynard MJ, Deng X, Wickiewicz TL, et al. The popliteofibular ligament – rediscovery of a key element in posterolateral knee stability. Am J Sports Med 1996;24:311–316

51. Sugita T, Amis AA. Anatomic and biomechanical study of the lateral collateral and popliteofibular ligaments. Am J Sports Med 2001;29:466–472

52. LaPrade RF, Bollom TS, Wentorf FA, Wills NJ, Meister K. Mechanical failure properties of the posterolateral structure of the knee. Am J Sports Med 2005;33:1386–1391

53. LaPrade RF, Ly TV, Wentorf FA, Engebretsen L. The posterolateral attachments of the knee: a qualitative and quantitative morphology of the fibular collateral ligament, popliteus tendon, popliteofibular ligament and lateral gastrocnemius tendon. Am J Sports Med 2003;31:854–860

54. LaPrade RF, Johansen S, Wentorf FA, Engebretsen L, Esterberg JL, Tso A. An analysis of an anatomic posterolateral knee reconstruction: an *in vitro* biomechanical study and development of a surgical technique. Am J Sports Med 2004;32:1405–1414

55. Wascher DC, Grauer JD, Markolf KL. Biceps tendon tenodesis for posterolateral instability of the knee. Am J Sports Med 1993;21:400–406

56. Albright JP, Brown AW. Management of chronic posterolateral rotatory instability of the knee: surgical technique for the posterolateral corner sling procedure. Instr Course Lect 1998;47:369–378

57. Clancy WG. Repair and reconstruction of the posterior cruciate ligament. In: Chapman M, ed. Operative Orthopaedics. Philadelphia: JB Lippincott, 1988:1651–1655

58. Clancy WG, Sutherland TB. Combined posterior cruciate ligament injuries. Clin Sports Med 1994;13:629–647

59. LaPrade RF, Wentorf FA, Crum JA. Assessment of healing of grade III posterolateral corner injuries: an *in vivo* model. J Orthop Res 2004;2:970–975

60. O'Brien SJ, Warren RF, Pavlov H, Panariello R, Wickiewicz TL. Reconstruction of the chronically insufficient anterior cruciate ligament with the central third of the patellar ligament. J Bone Joint Surg 1991;73A:278–286

61. Noyes FR, Barber-Westin SD, Hewitt TE. High tibial osteotomy and ligament reconstruction for varus angulated anterior cruciate ligament deficient knees. Am J Sports Med 2000;28:282–296

62. Noyes FR, Barber-Westin SD. Revision of anterior cruciate surgery with use of bone-patellar tendon-bone autogenous grafts. J Bone Joint Surg 2001;83A:1131–1143

7

Treatment of Posterolateral Knee Injuries

◆ Treatment of Grade 1 and Grade 2 Posterolateral Knee Injuries

The recommended treatment for grade 1 to 2, or partial, posterolateral knee injuries is almost always nonsurgical.[1] For isolated injuries, the treatment is usually immobilization of the knee in extension for 3 weeks to allow healing of the injured tissues. After 3 weeks, patients are allowed to work on regaining their range of motion. Depending on the amount of laxity present, patients may either bear weight in extension for mild injuries or may be non–weight-bearing for the initial 6 weeks while they are working on this rehabilitation protocol.

Patients begin a functional rehabilitation program starting at 6 weeks postinjury, working primarily on endurance exercises and avoiding any aggressive hamstring work at this time. The main exercises are an exercise bike, gentle leg presses to a maximum of 70 degrees of knee flexion, and a functional walking program. At 3 months postinjury, patients are allowed to increase their activities as tolerated based on their overall strength levels.

I recommend that patients who still have problems with pain or instability with this nonoperative treatment program should be reevaluated to determine if they have residual posterolateral instability that was either initially not recognized or did not heal. In addition, they should be carefully examined to make sure there is not another etiology of their symptoms that was not detected in the presence of their initial injury. My usual protocol in those instances, where it does appear that they have some residual laxity, is to place the patient into a medial compartment unloader brace and assess whether he or she has an improvement of the subjective symptoms, as well as to obtain bilateral varus stress radiographs to quantitate if the clinical exam of varus instability in fact may be underestimating the amount of true instability to varus opening. I have found the unloader brace to be very useful in determining those patients who I may have otherwise treated nonoperatively due to my inability to clinically detect the amount of knee instability that they may have with functional activities. Overall, these patients who I felt initially had only a grade 2 posterolateral corner knee injury that should be treated nonoperatively may in fact have had a grade III posterolateral corner knee injury, and all of these patients I treated who had alleviation of their symptoms in the unloader brace have had good functional results after a posterolateral knee reconstructive procedure. In general, my patients have not had any significant functional limitations with isolated popliteus complex injuries, which have an increase in posterolateral rotation in flexion primarily. Most patients with isolated posterolateral knee injuries have functional limitations when there is an increase in varus laxity.

Another etiology of functional limitation for these patients who may have these underlying injuries is the tears of the popliteomeniscal fascicles, and patients have associated pain from the resultant meniscal hypermobility. Some patients have increased lateral meniscal hypermobility when their popliteomeniscal fascicles are torn. As noted in Chapter 5, these patients are best diagnosed by putting the knee into a "figure-four" position to see if they have reproduction of their lateral compartment knee pain. In those patients that do, it may be appropriate to proceed with a diagnostic arthroscopy to determine if there is any lateral meniscal hypermobility to probing. If there is, it is recommended that an open or arthroscopic repair of the popliteomeniscal fascicles to the lateral meniscus be performed.[2]

Overall, the vast majority of patients who have isolated grade 1 or 2 posterolateral corner injuries recover well and return to full activities within 3 to 4 months after injury.

Combined Cruciate Ligament and Grade 1 to 2 Posterolateral Corner Injuries

Patients who are found to have grade 1 to 2 posterolateral corner injuries combined with an anterior cruciate ligament (ACL) or posterior cruciate ligament (PCL) tear need to be closely evaluated for the amount of instability that is caused by this combined injury pattern. In the vast majority of patients, it is recommended that the underlying cruciate ligament tear that has caused the instability be repaired or reconstructed and that the grade I to II posterolateral corner injury be treated nonoperatively and a protocol similar to that for isolated tears.

In those instances where the clinical exam may suggest increased laxity to a degree more than one would expect, it may be appropriate to obtain PCL stress radiographs or varus stress radiographs to determine the amount of instability. As was noted Chapter 6, increasing amounts of varus instability put extra stress on an ACL reconstructive graft, whereas both increased varus laxity and a combined posterolateral rotatory instability (coupled posterior and external rotation forces) place extra stress on a PCL reconstructive graft. In those instances where there is found to be increased amounts of varus laxity or where there are side-to-side differences in posterior translation of the PCL that on the stress radiographs exceeds 10 to 12 mm, it may be better to err on the side of being conservative and repair or reconstruct the posterolateral corner injury rather than treating it nonoperatively and running the risk of having the graft stretch out because of the extra forces on it due to this combined instability pattern.

◆ Surgical Treatment of Acute Grade III Isolated Posterolateral Knee Injuries

It has been well documented in the literature that grade 3 posterolateral corner injuries have a low likelihood of healing nonoperatively, and that surgical intervention is necessary to ensure the best clinical outcome.[3,4] It has also been demonstrated that the results of an acute repair are much improved compared with attempts at chronic repairs or reconstructive procedures.[5–7] Thus I recommend that an acute repair or reconstruction be performed in isolated grade 3 posterolateral corner injuries in all patients in whom it is feasible. In patients who have had degloving-type injuries of the skin over the posterolateral corner of their knee, open lacerations, or significant abrasions, it is more prudent to wait until these injuries heal prior to undergoing surgery. One issue in particular to be concerned about is subcutaneous degloving injuries. When a significant subcutaneous hematoma is found upon making the initial incision in these patients, there is a higher rate of infection due to the poorer blood supply to the skin flap. If this circumstance is encountered in an acute injury, it may be more prudent to abort the surgical treatment until the skin has a better chance to heal. In these and other instances in which there may be issues with healing, vascularity, or infection, waiting until these issues have resolved prior to proceeding with a surgical repair or reconstructive procedure is recommended.

Surgical repairs or reconstructions of grade III isolated posterolateral corner injuries should be done as soon as possible after injury, once it appears that the skin and soft tissues can safely undergo a surgical procedure. It has been the recommendation of the International Society of Arthroscopy, Knee Surgery, and Orthopaedic Sports Medicine (ISAKOS) Closed Knee Meeting on the Posterior Cruciate Ligament (and Posterolateral Knee) (Florence, Italy, November 2002) that these surgical procedures be performed within the first 2 weeks after a posterolateral injury. In some busy referral practices the patients may not come in until later. But I strongly recommend that these injuries should be addressed in the initial 2-week period after injury because the procedures are easier both on the patient and on the surgeon during this time interval. It is well recognized that approximately 3 weeks after injury, significant scar tissue planes can develop along the posterolateral knee that makes it very difficult to identify the superficial layer of the iliotibial band, the biceps femoris complex, and especially the common peroneal nerve. As I have reiterated to my residents and fellows in these circumstances, during this surgical approach, scar can look like nerve and the common peroneal nerve can look like scar, which requires meticulous attention and can increase the surgical time significantly while one is dissecting out the common peroneal nerve to allow it to be retracted out of the surgical field. In addition, operating soon after injury ensures that individual anatomic structures can be easily identified and can hold sutures sufficiently to allow for early protected range of motion after a repair. I have found that at about 3 weeks after injury, most of the main structures of the posterolateral knee do not hold sutures well and become necrotic, which makes it very difficult to allow for early range of motion after this type of repair. In addition, it becomes necessary to perform either augmentations or reconstructions of these structures after this point in time rather than repairing the native structures.

◆ Surgical Approach to the Posterolateral Knee

Proper intraoperative positioning is essential to performing these procedures. I use a sandbag taped to the bed, with a bump under the patient's hip, to allow the patient's knee to rest at about 70 degrees of knee flexion. It is important that the knee is balanced and can sit in this position without the need for an assistant to hold it. In this manner, the assistant can then concentrate on retracting skin and tissue flaps out of the operative field rather than also having to concentrate on balancing the knee (**Fig. 7–1**).

The skin incision consists of a lateral hockey-stick–shaped incision centered over Gerdy's tubercle. It follows the posterior border of the superificial layer of the iliotibial band and then continues distally over the anterior compartment of the knee parallel to the anterior tibial crest[8] (**Fig. 7–2**). The skin incision is drawn on the skin with a surgical marker with the knee flexed to about 70 degrees. I extend the knee after the skin incision is drawn to verify that the incision is basically a straight line in full extension.

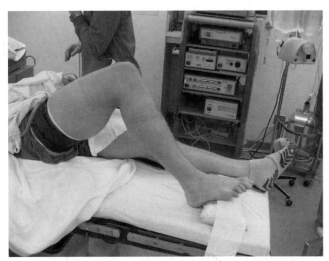

Figure 7–1   The ideal position of a patient's extremity on the examining table for a posterolateral knee surgical approach. A sandbag is taped to the bed, a bump is placed under the hip, and the knee is balanced at 70 degrees of knee flexion.

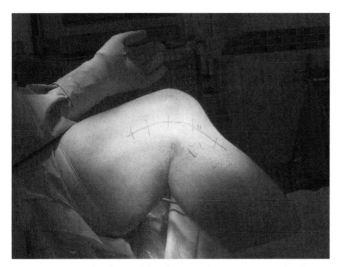

Figure 7–2   The lateral hockey-stick incision made for a posterolateral right knee surgical approach (fibular head outlined).

After the skin is incised, the subcutaneous tissues are then dissected down to expose the superficial layer of the iliotibial band. Sharp Sein (V. Mueller, Deerfield, Illinois) retractors are used by an assistant to apply tension at the skin margins to allow for improved identification of the subcutaneous tissues over the superficial layer of the iliotibial band. In the majority of acute cases, there may be some serous drainage from the subcutaneous tissues at the time of the skin incision. This usually occurs in combined posterolateral and cruciate ligament knee injuries, but I have also seen it in some isolated posterolateral knee injuries. This tissue edema indicates that there was a rather significant trauma over this part of the knee. I have not found these patients to have any increased problems with skin healing or postoperative drainage.

Once the superficial layer of the iliotibial band is identified, a posteriorly based subfascial flap is then meticulously dissected posteriorly over the musculature of the short head of the biceps femoris, down to the long head of the biceps femoris, and the proximal anterior compartment musculature of the leg (**Fig. 7–3**). In those instances where these structures are injured, the proximal part of the dissection is performed first to find the normal tissues and then performed distally to identify the avulsed, and possibly proximally retracted ends, of the biceps femoris complex off the fibula. It is important to identify the normal structures proximally and dissect distally to avoid injury to a potentially displaced course of the common peroneal nerve. After the skin flap is reflected, it is possible to view the entire lateral superficial fascia from the iliotibial band to the biceps femoris muscles.

In those patients with a large avulsion of structures off the femur, tibia, or fibula, I recommend that the injury planes be followed in the surgical dissection to identify the specific structures that have been damaged. In those instances in which the superficial layer of the iliotibial band and the biceps femoris complex are intact, I then proceed with performing a common peroneal neurolysis.

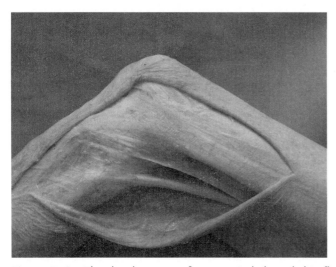

Figure 7–3 The development of a posteriorly based skin flap for the posterolateral knee approach (left knee).

I prefer to use an Adson (V. Mueller, Deerfield, Illinois) pointed hemostat to dissect along the soft tissue posterior to the long head of the biceps femoris to facilitate identifying the common peroneal nerve. These hemostats have a fine tip, which allows for meticulous dissection of the scar tissue away from the nerve without causing a lot of trauma to the surrounding tissues during this approach. In most of these acute injuries, there can be scar tissue formation already developing in this area, and it's important to go through the scar tissues slowly to make sure that one identifies the common peroneal nerve and document if there is hemorrhage, a bulbous appearance, or possibly an avulsion of the nerve due to the injury (**Fig. 7–4**). An assistant incises the tissues, layer by layer, that I lift up with the Atsen pointed hemostat during this part of the procedure. In most

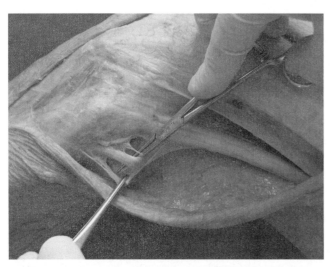

Figure 7–4 Common peroneal nerve neurolysis with hemostat around nerve, forceps holding surrounding aponeurotic tissue (left knee).

instances, the common peroneal nerve can be found by palpation, and sometimes the lateral band of adipose tissue that covers it can still be seen, to guide the surgeon to its course.

In those instances where there is such a significant amount of scar tissue that it is difficult to determine its course, I would then try either to find the common peroneal nerve more proximally to where it just crosses under the long head of the biceps femoris or to identify its course approximately 2 cm distal to the fibular head where it courses deep to the peroneal longus musculature and then follow its course proximally.

The standard deep approach incisions include two fascial incisions, a horizontal splitting incision in the anterior arm of the long head of the biceps femoris, and a vertical lateral capsular incision. It is important to use only those deep approach incisions that are felt to be necessary based on the location of pain or swelling, arthroscopic or magnetic resonance imaging (MRI) identification of a specific injury, or the plane of injury identified during the surgical approach to this area. These incisions have been found to allow for consistent access to all of the individual anatomic structures of the posterolateral knee.

The first fascial incision is performed concurrently with a common peroneal nerve neurolysis to allow for retraction of the nerve and to gain access to the fibular styloid attachments and posterior aspect of the knee. I almost always perform a common peroneal nerve neurolysis to gain access to the structures over the posterolateral corner of the knee. I have never had a case of postoperative neuropraxia in a normal-appearing nerve or of pain or dysesthesias developing due to scarring of the nerve at any time postoperatively. Once I have dissected out the common peroneal nerve sufficiently, I place a small Penrose drain around it to allow it to be gently retracted out of the field while we are working in that area. I prefer not to attach a hemostat to the Penrose drain because it could inadvertently result in the nerve being put under traction by an unwary or tired assistant while I am working on other associated knee injuries. I also like to have the scrub nurse or an assistant hold the foot at this point to see if the nerve is being irritated during the neurolysis. In those cases when it is very irritable and there is significant ankle dorsiflexion firing, I slow down the nerve dissection and try to not cause further nerve irritation.

The interval between the lateral gastrocnemius tendon/muscle complex and the soleus muscle is then entered by blunt dissection with one's fingers. Through this interval, one can palpate the popliteofibular ligament and its attachment on the posteromedial aspect of the fibular styloid, the musculotendinous junction of the popliteus, as well as all the way over to the PCL attachment facet of the tibia (**Fig. 7–5**). In cases where there is significant scar tissue in this interval, an Adson pointed hemostat can be utilized to open a window in this scar tissue to allow one's fingers to enter this interval. This surgical approach allows one to gain access to the posteromedial aspect of the fibular styloid when the popliteofibular ligament needs to be repaired or reconstructed, as well as to the coronary ligament to the posterior horn of the lateral meniscus when this also needs to be repaired acutely.

The second, and main, fascial splitting incision is performed through the superficial layer of the iliotibial band. This incision is performed from just proximal to the supracondylar flare of the femur, in line with the fibers of the superficial

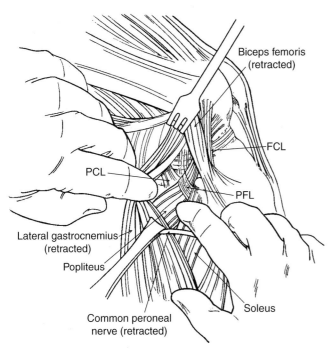

Figure 7–5 The surgical development of the interval between the lateral gastrocnemius and soleus muscles. Through this interval, one's finger can palpate for a tear of the popliteofibular ligament (PFL), the popliteus tendon, and the posterior cruciate ligament (PCL) at its attachment on the PCL facet on the posterior aspect of the tibia (lateral view, right knee). FCL, fibular collateral ligament.

layer of the iliotibial band, and extends distally through this superficial layer to Gerdy's tubercle **(Fig. 7–6)**. I usually place a small mosquito hemostat under the superficial layer of the iliotibial band as I make this incision so that I do not harm any deeper structures while incising it. This splitting incision allows the superficial

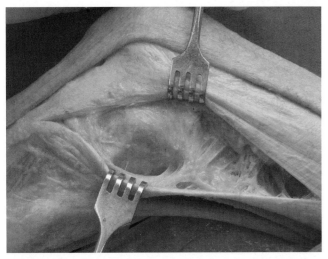

Figure 7–6 The iliotibial band splitting incision, left knee (superficial layer held in retractors).

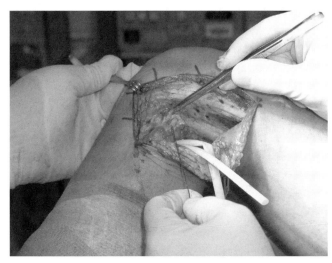

Figure 7–7 Entering through the biceps bursa, the fibular collateral ligament is identified and a traction suture is placed into the ligament (lateral view, left knee).

layer of the iliotibial band to be retracted both anteriorly and posteriorly, and one can then gain access to the attachment sites of the fibular collateral ligament, lateral gastrocnemius tendon, and popliteus tendon on the femur, as well as to the mid-third lateral capsular ligament and posterolateral capsule of the knee.

A small horizontal incision is then made through the anterior arm of the long head of the biceps femoris, where it crosses the fibular collateral ligament, about 1 cm proximal to the fibular head. This incision enters the biceps bursa and allows for identification of the attachment site of the fibular collateral ligament on the lateral aspect of the fibular head. The fibular attachment of the fibular collateral ligament is easily identified through this incision (**Fig. 7–7**). I place a small suture into the fibular collateral ligament and tug on it at this point to identify any significant laxity, as well as to identify its attachment site on the femur in those cases where it has not been completely torn. The tension applied through this traction stitch usually allows visualizing the entire course of the fibular collateral ligament at this point. The biceps bursa covers about 25% of the fibular collateral ligament, and I have found many distal injuries to be easily identified through this interval. In addition, in those instances where it has been avulsed off the femur and it is very difficult to identify it through scar tissue formation proximally, utilizing the suture to tug on the fibular collateral ligament makes it easier to identify its course proximally and to minimize dissection to find its course.

A less commonly used fascial splitting incision is performed in the interval between the posterior border of the iliotibial band and the short head of the biceps femoris. Through this incision, one can see the attachment site of the anterior arm of the short head of the biceps femoris as well as attachment site of the lateral capsule on the tibia.[8,9] Although we did use it as a major incision to gain access to posterolateral knee injuries in the past, I rarely use it currently as I have found the other incisions allow me to gain access to all of the injured structures as my experience and familiarity with these injury patterns grow. I have found this incision to be primarily useful in acute cases where there has been a tibial-based lateral avulsion injury of the meniscotibial portion of the mid-third lateral capsular ligament and a concurrent tear of the anterior arm of the short head of the biceps femoris. This bony or soft tissue Segond avulsion variant is usually easily identified on axial or coronal MRI images.[10]

At this time, I have usually identified the injury pattern of most of the individual structures of the posterolateral corner of the knee. I also usually have not used a tourniquet because there is usually little bleeding encountered with this approach in the acute injury phase.

Arthroscopic Evaluation of the Lateral Compartment of the Knee

Once these structures have been identified, I perform a diagnostic arthroscopy of the knee to assess the intraarticular status of the posterolateral corner. Standard arthroscopic portals are placed to allow for fluid inflow and outflow. The lateral working portal is placed adjacent to the patellar tendon, with the medial arthroscopic portal placed just medial to the patellar tendon and at the joint line. A 30-degree arthroscope is utilized in this instance.

The first lateral compartment observation is to determine the amount of lateral compartment opening. In my series, I have found that there is always greater than 1 cm of lateral compartment opening when there is a grade 3 posterolateral corner injury present,[11] and the posterior horn of the lateral meniscus is well visualized. During this portion of the arthroscopy it is important to determine whether this is a meniscofemoral- or a meniscotibial-based injury. Placing a varus stress on the knee with an arthroscope in the lateral compartment will allow one to see whether the meniscus moves with the femur or with the tibia, and one can focus the further surgical incisions based on this observation. If the meniscus stays with the tibia, it usually indicates a femoral-based avulsion or intrasubstance stretch injury of the popliteus tendon and probably also the fibular collateral ligament. When the meniscus stays with the femur, it usually indicates a significant lateral capsular or Segond-variant soft tissue or bony avulsion pattern.[10,12] One can also determine the amount of injury that is present and start to think about postoperative rehabilitation limitations to maximize healing and outcome.

An arthroscopic probe is utilized to probe the circumference of the lateral meniscus to determine if there is any meniscal hypermobility or tearing **(Fig. 7–8)**. Most of the time, there are either no tears or a peripheral tear of the lateral meniscus. I have had to perform a lateral meniscectomy most commonly with combined ACL and posterolateral knee injuries. In addition, the integrity of the coronary ligament to the posterior horn of the lateral meniscus is assessed to determine if a direct open repair, through the interval between the lateral gastrocnemius and the soleus, will be necessary during the open repair portion of the procedure. Once the lateral meniscus has been totally evaluated, the 30-degree arthroscope is placed in the lateral gutter with the knee flexed at about 30 degrees and in slight valgus to visualize the popliteus attachment on the femur as well as to assess the integrity of the popliteomeniscal fascicles. In general, I have found that the popliteus tendon tends to sit right up against the capsule and not to retract distally when it has been torn off the femur. To

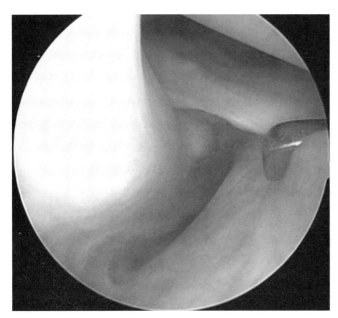

Figure 7–8   Probing for lateral meniscal pathology peripherally for any laxity at the popliteal hiatus (normal popliteomeniscal fascicles, right knee).

properly evaluate the femoral attachment of the popliteus tendon at this time, one must observe it while both an internal and external rotation torque is applied to the tibia. I have found the femoral attachment to look fairly normal in some circumstances when first inserting the arthroscope into the lateral compartment, and then found it to completely disengage off its femoral attachment site with application of an external rotation force. In my study, I found it to be torn off the femur in 33% of patients with a grade 3 posterolateral corner injury. The rest of the injuries were intrasubstance stretch or musculotendinous junction avulsion injuries. In addition, up to 75% of patients have some tearing of the anteroinferior popliteomeniscal fascicle to the lateral meniscus. The amount of hypermobility caused by tearing of the structure can be assessed by probing the lateral meniscus at this location. As I noted in the section on clinically relevant biomechanics, the anteroinferior popliteomeniscal fascicle is the larger meniscal attachment fascicle and it seems to provide the most stability to the lateral meniscus. It is important to document potential lateral meniscal hypermobility due to tears of this structure by directly probing it at this time.

In those instances where the popliteus tendon has been found to be avulsed off the femur, or if there is any lateral meniscal hypermobility because of the tear of the popliteomeniscal fascicles, a lateral capsular arthrotomy incision is then made after the arthroscopic evaluation of the knee has been completed to allow access to repair these structures.

Once the lateral compartment has been assessed for injuries, and other intraarticular structure injuries are resected, repaired, or reconstructed, attention can be turned to the repair or reconstruction of the torn posterolateral structures.

The lateral capsular arthrotomy incision is made by retracting the edges of the superficial layer of the iliotibial band both anteriorly and posteriorly at the

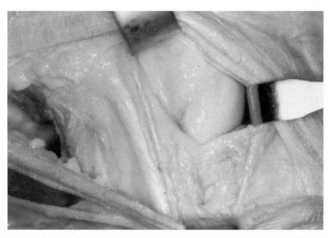

Figure 7–9   Lateral capsular arthrotomy incision. The popliteus tendon, popliteomeniscal fascicles, lateral meniscus, and inferior lateral genicular artery are identified through this approach (retractors holding incised meniscofemoral capsule) (right knee).

lateral joint line. A vertical incision is then made through the meniscofemoral portion of the mid-third lateral capsular ligament, approximately 1 cm anterior to the course of the fibular collateral ligament **(Fig. 7–9)**. With the knee flexed to 70 degrees, the normal course of the fibular collateral ligament is parallel to and in line with the fibular shaft.[8] In those knees in which the fibular collateral ligament is not well identified, due to injury, when one is tugging on the suture placed into the fibular collateral ligament through the biceps bursa distally, the knife handle can be placed along the course of the shaft of the fibula in this location, with the knee flexed to 70 degrees, and the incision made 1 cm anterior to this fibular shaft **(Fig. 7–10)**. Of course, it is important to verify that the torn

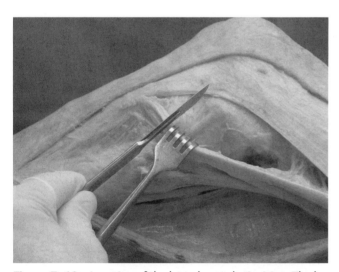

Figure 7–10   Location of the lateral capsular incision. The knee is flexed to 70 degrees, the knife blade is placed along the fibular shaft, and the incision is made 1 cm anterior to this landmark (left knee).

fibular collateral ligament is not caught in scar tissue when this incision is made so it is not inadvertently cut during this approach.

The lateral capsular incision has to be made carefully so the deep structures are not cut. The incision in this location should be just slightly anterior to the popliteus tendon attachment on the femur. Distal extension of the incision is then performed down to the level of the lateral meniscus. It is important to make sure that one does not incise into the substance of the lateral meniscus while making this incision by holding one edge of the capsule away from the lateral meniscus with a surgical forceps to obtain optimal visualization. In addition, it is important to coagulate or ligate the inferior lateral genicular artery where it crosses within the substance of the lateral capsule at the level of the lateral meniscus at this location to prevent significant postoperative bleeding. Sharp Sein retractors can then be placed into the incised edges of the lateral capsule and retracted apart to allow for identification of the popliteus tendon, lateral meniscus, and the popliteomeniscal fascicles. A whip stitch can be placed in the substance of the popliteus tendon at this time for performing a recess procedure if it has been torn off its femoral attachment. In addition, a direct repair of the popliteomeniscal fascicles back to the lateral meniscus can also be performed.

Once these various injuries have been identified in the acute situation, attention is now turned toward repair of specific anatomic structures or groups of structures to their native attachment sites. In addition, if these have been found to be nonrepairable tears, such as midsubstance tears of the fibular collateral ligament or popliteus tendon, plans are set into motion to use local uninjured tissue, hamstring autografts, or allografts to reconstruct these structures. The necessary instruments for these respective procedures should be obtained (if they have not been obtained already) at this time.

Structures That Attach to the Fibular Head and Styloid

Avulsions of the popliteofibular ligament, the direct arms of the short and long heads of the biceps femoris, the anterior arm of the long head of the biceps femoris, and the fibular collateral ligament off the fibular head and styloid should be repaired directly back to their anatomic attachment sites. Although many of my older colleagues perform a direct suture repair of these avulsed structures through drill holes, I have found that the use of suture anchors in these locations has many advantages. First, multiple suture anchors can be placed in the fibular head and styloid to repair all the specific avulsed structures back to their attachment sites (**Fig. 7–11**). Second, because the suture anchors can be placed directly at the attachment sites of these individual structures, the structures can be placed back in their native location and a strong secure fixation can be obtained. This step is very important because it can allow for early protected range of motion without any increased risk of stretching out of the surgical repair.

Structures That Attach to the Lateral Tibia

The main posterolateral structures that attach to the lateral aspect of the tibia include the anterior arm of the short head of the biceps femoris, the meniscotibial

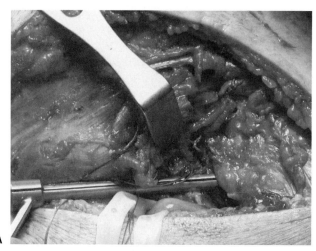
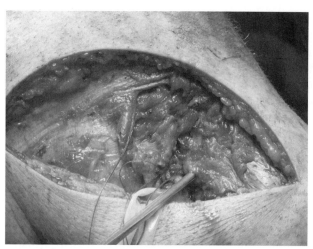

Figure 7–11   Placement of suture anchors in the fibular styloid **(A)** and head **(B)** to repair an avulsed long head of the biceps femoris, short head of the biceps femoris, popliteofibular ligament, and fibular collateral ligament anatomically (right knee).

portion of the mid-third lateral capsular ligament, the capsulo-osseous layer of the iliotibial band, and the superficial layer of the iliotibial band's attachment site at Gerdy's tubercle. In most instances, the structures tend to avulse or peel directly off the bone in a bony or soft tissue Segond-type avulsion injury.

I have found that the metaphyseal bone in the tibia in this location is usually soft and often does not sufficiently hold a suture anchor in most instances. Well-placed suture anchors in this location can sometimes be tugged directly out of the bone when one attempts to verify good secure purchase of the anchor in the bone. For this reason, I often use a No. 5 nonabsorbable suture on a large needle that is placed directly into the bone to repair these structures back to the anatomic locations. The entry and exit sites of the needle are about 1.5 to 2 cm apart in these instances. Because it may be difficult to place the meniscotibial portion of the mid-third lateral capsular ligament back exactly along this location when there is a large peeling off of the lateral soft tissues, suture anchors just distal to the articular margin of the tibia in this location may be placed, in addition to the direct suture repair further distal along the lateral tibia to bone, to obtain an anatomic repair at this location. Suture anchors placed right at the distal margin of the articular cartilage hold well in this location, but they need to be aimed so the tips of the anchors do not engage the subchondral bone and overlying articular cartilage **(Fig. 7–12)**.

In a similar fashion, suture anchors are usually necessary to repair the iliotibial band back to Gerdy's tubercle when it is avulsed off. In addition, injuries at this location are usually combined with a midsubstance injury that may need a spanning soft tissue portion of an Achilles allograft or autogenous hamstring graft to cover the area of the defect. In most instances where there has been a midstance injury to the superficial layer of the iliotibial band, a patch of allograft or autograft tissue must be sewn in place both to fill in the defect and to reinforce the remaining rim of injured tissue from these severe injuries.

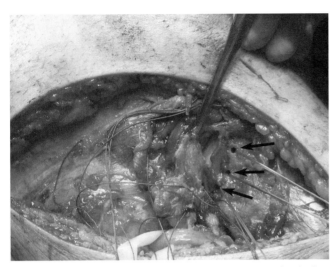

Figure 7–12   Repair of lateral capsular avulsions back directly to bone with suture anchors (arrows) just distal to articular margin (lateral view, right knee).

◆ Femoral-Based Posterolateral Knee Injuries

The posterolateral structures that can be torn off the femur for these injuries include the lateral gastrocnemius tendon, the meniscofemoral portion of the posterior capsule, the meniscofemoral portion of the mid-third lateral capsular ligament, the fibular collateral ligament, and the popliteus tendon. Injuries to these structures can readily be visualized through the iliotibial band fascial splitting incision. Suture anchors can be readily used to reattach the lateral gastrocnemius tendon and the portions of the posterior and lateral capsule to their anatomic femoral attachment sites when they are torn at these locations. However, I have not found the use of suture anchors to be secure enough for the avulsions of the fibular collateral ligament and the popliteus tendon off the femur to allow for early range of motion. It has been almost a decade since I attempted this type of direct anatomic repair because I found that I just couldn't make the fibular collateral ligament or the popliteus tendon tight enough against the bone to feel confident that it would heal in this location; gapping of the attachment of these structures was often visualized when a range of motion was assessed.

As I noted elsewhere,[9] I have used an adaptation of Roli Jakob's chronic popliteus tendon recess procedure to perform a recess procedure of the fibular collateral ligament or popliteus tendon when it has been torn off the femur in acute injuries.[13]

Popliteus Tendon or Fibular Collateral Ligament Femoral Recess Procedure

In acute instances, the recess procedure is performed by first placing a nonabsorbable No. 2 suture through the avulsed end of the fibular collateral ligament or the popliteus tendon in a whip stitch fashion to obtain a secure purchase. I

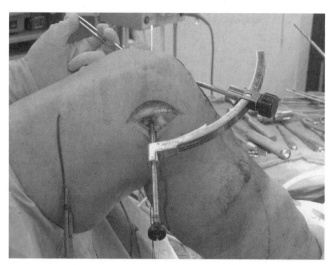

Figure 7–13   An acute fibular collateral ligament recess procedure with Beath pin placement, demonstrating its course is placed proximal to the adductor tubercle and not through the notch (right knee).

prefer not to use No. 5 sutures as I have found them to be too bulky and they commonly break when I pull them transversely across the femur with an eyelet passing pin. I then tug on this repair to make sure it is secure enough to allow for fixation as well as to verify that there is no midsubstance injury of the ligament or tendon that was not recognized. In addition, it allows me to determine if there will be enough length to be able to pull the end of the tendon into the tunnel for the recess procedure.

Once the passing stitch has been placed and it has been verified that there is sufficient length on both ends of the suture to allow it to be passed through the femur and tied over a button medially, I then use a cruciate ligament guide to place an eyelet-tipped pin through the exact attachment site of the fibular collateral ligament or popliteus tendon and have it exit the femur medially. When placing this eyelet-tipped pin it is important to be sure that the pin comes out proximal to the medial epicondyle and adductor tubercle region **(Fig. 7–13)**. Otherwise, one runs the risk of passing the recess procedure suture through the intercondylar notch. In addition, this pin should come out anterior to the adductor magnus tendon. I usually make a horizontal incision first, prior to placing the cruciate ligament guide on the distal femur in this location, to make sure that I'm coming out in the desired location. This horizontal incision is made slightly proximal to the course of the medial patellofemoral ligament and along the distal border of the vastus medialis obliquus muscle. The incision is extended deeper to between the vastus medialis obliquus muscle and the medial patellofemoral ligament to gain access to the femur. The vastus medialis obliquus muscle is then retracted proximally to allow the passing sutures and surgical button to be tied deep to the muscle fibers at this location.

Once the eyelet-tipped passing pin has been placed, a 5- or 6-mm cannulated reamer is then placed over it and reamed to a depth of 1 cm **(Fig. 7–14)**. The passing sutures in the end of the fibular collateral ligament, or the popliteus

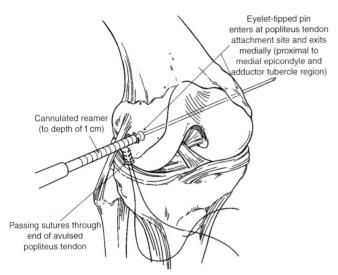

Figure 7–14 Popliteus tendon recess procedure. Illustration demonstrating reaming over the Beath pin, sutures already in the ends of the torn popliteus tendon, and the guide pin in place to pull the sutures medially to tie over a button on the femur. This will recess the end of the torn popliteus into the reamed tunnel (right knee).

tendon, are then placed into the eyelet-tipped pin and the pin and passing sutures are pulled out medially. I then verify by pulling on the sutures that I can pull the avulsed structure up into the tunnel created by the reamer in full knee extension. Once I can verify this, the ends of the passing sutures are then placed through a surgical button, which is placed deep to the vastus medialis obliquus muscle, directly against the medial cortex of the femur, and the sutures are tied down in this location with tension to pull the avulsed ligament or tendon up into the recess hole (**Fig. 7–15**). I prefer to tie the recess procedure sutures near

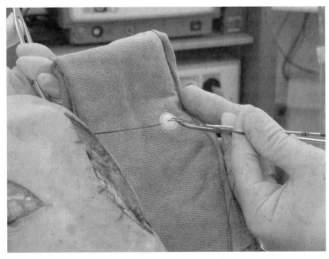

Figure 7–15 The sutures of a popliteus recess procedure to be tied over a button medially (right knee).

or at full extension so I know that I can obtain full knee extension immediately after surgery.

I have been very impressed by how secure this type of direct repair can be and I have confidence in allowing patients to initiate early motion after a recess procedure. I have not had any problems with laxity developing in these patients if all the above steps are closely followed.

Intrasubstance Injuries

The main soft tissues that can be repaired directly with intrasubstance injuries are the popliteomeniscal fascicles and the coronary ligament to the lateral meniscus. Other minor soft tissues that should be repaired in acute injuries include the lateral aponeurotic attachments from the biceps femoris muscles to the fibular collateral ligament and intrasubstance injuries of the deep and cap-sulo-osseous layers of the iliotibial band off the femur.

The popliteomeniscal fascicles can be repaired through the mid-third lateral capsular arthrotomy incision. A direct suture repair of the anteroinferior and posterosuperior popliteomeniscal fascicles can be made to the popliteus tendon through this location. I prefer to use a direct horizontal mattress suture repair with a nonabsorbable 0 suture so that I know that early motion can be initiated after this repair.

Tears of the coronary ligament to the posterior horn of the lateral meniscus are much more difficult to access. It is important to make sure that the lateral gastrocnemius is properly retracted posteriorly when using this approach to protect the neurovascular bundle. In those cases where the tourniquet is not in-flated, I would recommend that one palpate the popliteal artery to verify its location prior to suturing the meniscus back to the avulsed capsule.

A direct suture repair of a coronary ligament tear is performed by passing the suture needle through the popliteal aponeurosis to the lateral meniscus, into the substance of the lateral meniscus, and then down into the distal tibial attachment site of the coronary ligament (**Fig. 7–16**). I make sure that the assistant is retract-ing the lateral gastrocnemius and neurovascular bundle posteriorly during this time. I attempt to place the curved needle into the lateral meniscus directly on my first pass and then to have it pass down into the more distal portion of the coro-nary ligament. A second free needle driver may be used to grasp the tip of the nee-dle as it exits the posterior tissues, while the original needle driver holds the base of the needle in place. This helps to make sure the needles do not get lost in the posterior soft tissues. In that regard, I am certain that I can pull the lateral menis-cus back toward the tibia and prevent any residual laxity of this structure, which could result in hyperextension of the knee or hypermobility of the posterior horn of the lateral meniscus. Multiple sutures along the course of this tear should be placed and then tied with the knee flexed to be able to obtain a good secure repair.

Acute Reconstruction of the Popliteus Tendon with an Autogenous Hamstring Graft

Midsubstance tears of the popliteus tendon or musculotendinous junction avulsions are usually not amenable to a direct suture repair. In these instances,

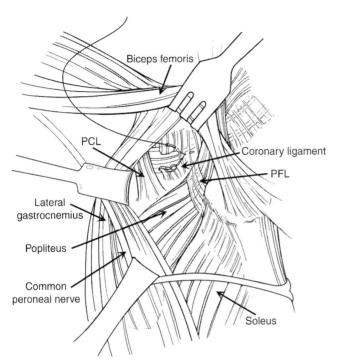

Figure 7–16 A coronary ligament repair of the lateral meniscus performed through the interval between the lateral gastrocnemius tendon and the soleus muscles. A direct repair is performed with a suture, grabbing the lateral meniscus with a needle (lateral meniscus ghosted in) (lateral view, right knee).

in the acute situation, I usually harvest an ipsilateral semitendinosus tendon and use it to reconstruct the popliteus tendon. In this instance, a small 2- to 3-cm-long vertical incision is placed just distal and medial to the tibial tubercle to identify the gracilis and semitendinosus attachments on the tibia. Once the proximal aspect of the pes anserine attachment sites have been identified, an incision is made through the sartorius fascia to identify the semitendinosus tendon in this location and then it is harvested using a hamstring stripper. I prefer to leave the gracilis in place to avoid any potential saphenous nerve irritation and to obtain the thicker of the two main hamstring grafts. The tendon is then taken down off the tibia, and the muscle that is obtained as part of the harvesting is then dissected off. Both ends of the semitendinosus tendon are then tubulized, using a No. 2 and No. 5 suture, to allow it to be utilized to reconstruct the popliteus tendon.

The femoral attachment site of an acute reconstruction of the popliteus tendon is performed in a similar fashion as the recess procedure. However, I attempt to place at least 25 mm of the hamstring tendon in the femoral tunnel in this location. It can be either fixed in the femur in this location with a bioabsorbable screw or tied medially over a surgical button using a recess type fixation. I should note that if one uses a bioabsorbable screw in this location, the tunnels should be tapped prior to placing the interference screw as the bone is quite hard in this location. Once the graft has been fixed in the femur, it is then passed distally through the popliteal hiatus to exit into the space between the lateral gastrocnemius and soleus muscles at the musculotendinous junction of the popliteus. A second tunnel is then drilled in the tibia to allow for fixation of this graft. There is a small sulcus at the musculotendinous junction in the tibia that can be palpated,[14] which is where the tunnel site should exit. A cruciate ligament guide can be used to drill this tunnel. The entry site on the tibia is best placed just distal and medial to Gerdy's tubercle. The tibia is flat in this location and it's easy to pass a guide pin here. Guide pins that are placed lateral to this location commonly drift along the lateral aspect of the tibia and a less than ideal bone tunnel may be drilled. A guide pin is drilled from anterior to posterior at this location that will come out posteriorly on the tibia at the musculotendinous junction. It is important to place a posterior retractor in this interval to protect the posterior structures when the guide pin exits. A 7- or 8-mm reamer is then utilized to ream this tunnel. Once the tunnel has been reamed, attention is now turned toward passing the graft out anteriorly from its posterior entry point at the popliteus musculotendinous junction to the anterior tunnel aperture, which is located just distomedial to Gerdy's tubercle.

If there is any native popliteus muscle or if the popliteus musculotendinous junction is still intact in this location, I attempt to weave the graft through this substance and then to pass it out anteriorly on the tibia. The knee is placed in 60 degrees of flexion and neutral rotation while the graft is pulled anteriorly and fixed on the tibia with a bioabsorbable screw. I do not attempt to internally rotate the tibia during fixation as I am concerned it may overconstrain the knee and prevent normal physiologic external rotation. The metaphyseal bone in this location is usually much softer than in the femur and I have not found that I have had to use a tap for the bioabsorbable screw. I also use a small bone staple to back up the bioabsorbable screw in this location, directly over the flat spot distal and medial to Gerdy's tubercle, for fixation (**Fig. 7–17**).

Acute Reconstruction of the Fibular Collateral Ligament

Midsubstance tears of the fibular collateral ligament can sometimes be repaired and augmented with a strip of the long head of the biceps femoris as a graft. It is important to recognize that this type of surgical repair can only be performed when there is no injury to the long head of the biceps tendon. In those instances where the long head of the biceps tendon can be utilized to supplement a tear of the fibular collateral ligament, a distally based strip of tendon is harvested. It is important to measure the distance between the lateral aspect of the fibular head and its attachment site on the femur to make sure that one obtains a long enough strip of tendon to perform the reconstruction. In most instances, this appears to be about 70 mm long. I recommend separating the tendon longitudinally, prior to amputating it proximally, as this allows for easier handling of this band of harvested tissue. Once this distal-based strip of tendon has been obtained, it needs to be attached on the fibula close to the normal attachment site of the fibular collateral ligament (**Fig. 7–18**). To do this, a suture anchor is placed at this location and it is tied into the apex of this tendon strip to post it at this location. If one relies solely on the soft tissue fixation of the biceps distally to hold this graft, it will not be an anatomic reconstruction

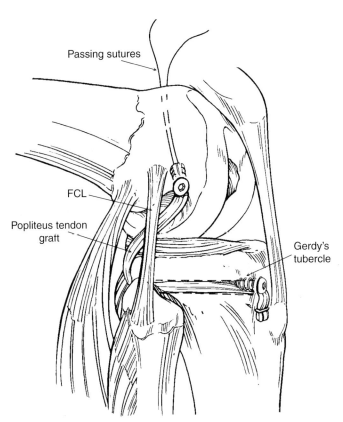

Passing sutures

FCL

Popliteus tendon
graft

Gerdy's
tubercle

Figure 7–17   Acute popliteus tendon reconstruction using a hamstring graft. Illustration demonstrating the hamstring pulled up into the femoral tunnel and fixed in place with a bioabsorbable screw, wrapped around the musculotendinous junction of the popliteus complex, and pulled out anteriorly through the tibial tunnel and fixed in place with a screw and staple (right knee).

as the anterior arm of the long biceps attaches to the anterior aspect of the fibular head. Passing stitches can then be placed into the proximal aspect of this strip of biceps and then it can be either attached to the femur in a recess type procedure or directly repaired to bone with suture anchors and sutures along the course of the native fibular collateral ligament to supplement an intrasubstance injury.

In those instances where the biceps femoris is also injured, which usually is more common than when it is not in this circumstance, the fibular collateral ligament can be anatomically reconstructed using one of the hamstring tendons. In a similar fashion to how a semitendinosus graft was described to be harvested for the popliteus tendon, it is also harvested and two sutures are used to tubulize each end of the graft to allow it to be passed into the femoral tunnel with the use of an eyelet tipped pin. The femoral attachment site of the fibular collateral ligament is identified and a 7-mm reamer is used to drill a 20- to 25-mm deep tunnel over the eyelet-tipped passing pin in this location. A bioabsorbable screw is usually utilized to hold it in its location. Once again, the screw hole should be tapped prior to inserting the bioabsorbable screw because

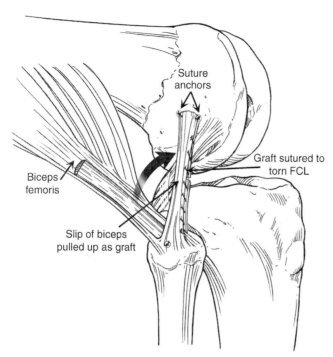

Figure 7–18   Illustration of a right knee demonstrating the use of a distal-based lateral slip of the long head of the biceps tendon to augment a repair of a midsubstance fibular collateral ligament tear. Note: One suture anchor is used to post the biceps tendon to the fibula. The other suture anchors are placed along the femur at the anatomic attachment site of the fibular collateral ligament for this augmentation repair (lateral view, right knee).

of the hard nature of the femoral bone in this location. To accomplish this without completely removing the eyelet pin, the eyelet pin can be pulled medially until it is recessed into the femoral tunnel and then pulled back laterally once the tunnel has been tapped. Once the graft has been secured in the femoral tunnel, the passing sutures can be cut off medially.

A second tunnel is now drilled through the fibular head and the styloid. The tunnel enters the lateral aspect of the fibular head at the exact attachment site of the fibular collateral ligament in this location. The tunnel then exits through the posterior aspect of the fibular styloid; make sure that it does not exit through or damage the popliteofibular ligament fibular attachment site. One also needs to make sure that the entry point of this tunnel is drilled distal enough on the lateral aspect of the fibula so that it does not break out the proximal aspect of the fibular head. It is also important to aim this tunnel slightly distal and central on the fibular styloid so the popliteofibular ligament is not injured at its exit site. A 6- or 7-mm cannulated reamer is used to drill a tunnel in this location. In patients with soft bone, a smaller tunnel may be drilled and tunnel dilators used to enlarge the tunnel. Once it has been drilled, the graft utilized to reconstruct the fibular collateral ligament is then passed under the superficial layer of the iliotibial band and the lateral aponeurosis to the long head of the biceps femoris and passed through the tunnel and then pulled back

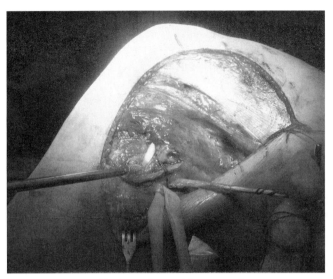

Figure 7–19 A fibular collateral ligament hamstring autograft reconstruction. The graft is placed in the femoral tunnel and fixed with a bioabsorbable screw. The graft passes under the superficial layer of the iliotibial band and the lateral aponeurotic layer of the long head of the biceps femoris. The tunnel is placed through the anatomic attachment site laterally on the fibular head for the fibular collateral ligament and exits posteriorly to avoid the popliteofibular ligament attachment. The graft is then tied back on itself, after it is fixed in the fibular tunnel with a bioabsorbable screw (left knee).

upon itself. I then place the knee in 30 degrees of knee flexion, in neutral rotation, with a valgus force on the knee to reduce any increase in varus opening. Bioabsorbable screws are then placed into the fibular head to secure the graft at this location. I have not found that I need to tap for the bioabsorbable screw placement in the fibular head. I then verify that the varus instability at 30 degrees of knee flexion has been eliminated over the side of the table once the fibular screw has been secured. Once this is confirmed, I bring the graft from its posterior location and tie it back on itself at the lateral fibular location, with horizontal mattress 0-Vicryl or nonabsorbable sutures. This serves to supplement and back up the bioabsorbable screw fixation **(Fig. 7–19)**.

In those instances where both of these structures have been torn in their midsubstance and cannot be repaired, a direct anatomic reconstruction using an Achilles tendon allograft is then performed. This technique is described in detail in the section on chronic reconstructions that follows.

Until just recently, no surgical technique has been developed to treat posterolateral knee instability with an anatomic reconstruction of the three main static stabilizing structures of the posterolateral knee: the fibular collateral ligament, the popliteus tendon, and the popliteofibular ligament. Surgical treatment of chronic grade III posterolateral knee injuries has included various reconstructions, tenodesis procedures, osteotomies, and advancement procedures for chronic injuries, for example, the fibular collateral ligament reconstruction,[15,16] femoral bone block advancements,[17-20] biceps femoris tenodesis,[21-24] valgus high tibial osteotomies,[9] popliteus tendon and popliteofibular ligament reconstructions using split patellar tendon grafts,[16] popliteus recess procedures,[13] and central slip iliotibial band or biceps femoris grafts.[16,25,26] Although these surgical techniques may provide varying degrees of varus, external rotation, and coupled posterolateral motion stability to knees with these posterolateral injuries, none of them anatomically reconstructs these three main static stabilizers by reproducing the normal anatomy. In addition, there has been a paucity of in vitro biomechanical studies for these described posterolateral reconstruction procedures.[24] I believe that an anatomic reconstruction of the posterolateral knee will ultimately result in improved objective motion stability and patient function compared with these nonanatomic techniques. Through our quantitative anatomy work, we developed a reconstructive technique that is outlined in the following pages. In addition, prior to trialing this in patients, we performed a thorough biomechanical analysis to prove that it does restore stability to knees that have these injuries (see Chapter 6).

◆ The Development and Evolution of a Surgical Technique for Midsubstance or Chronic Tears of the Main Structures of the Posterolateral Knee

I owe a lot to Glenn "Corky" Terry, Champ Baker, and the late Jack Hughston for their guidance in the early part of my sports medicine training at the Hughston Clinic in Columbus, Georgia, in posterolateral knee injuries. They recognized my enthusiasm for attacking this relative "black box" portion of sports medicine and had many discussions with me about how to proceed with an academic career. I took their discussions and recommendations to heart in trying to develop my strategy and research laboratory to help in the understanding and treatment of posterolateral knee injuries. They recommended to me that I should look at this area as a pyramid and attempt to build the base of the pyramid with a strong foundation of the understanding of the anatomy of the posterolateral knee, and follow that up with studies on biomechanics and the diagnosis of these injuries. In the course of doing this, I recognized that our sports medicine profession's evolution in the treatment of these injuries was very similar to the history and treatment for both anterior cruciate and PCL injuries. Our profession's early attempt at ACL reconstructions were primarily extraarticular sling procedures, whereas reconstructions of the PCL were also relatively nonanatomic. One published study used the medial meniscus to reconstruct the ACL in the clinical situation.[27] I performed a thorough search of this cruciate ligament surgical history and recognized the strong parallel to what I was seeing in the treatment of posterolateral knee injuries. I found that most of the procedures described for treating the posterolateral knee were nonanatomic, or sling type, procedures and that there weren't any quantitative studies on the anatomy of the posterolateral knee that could be utilized to further spring into developing an anatomic posterolateral knee reconstruction procedure. A careful analysis now demonstrates that the best clinical and objective results for cruciate ligament reconstruction grafts reproduce the normal anatomy of either the anterior[28–33] or posterior[34] cruciate ligaments.

By this time, I had performed several qualitative anatomy studies and had further developed a fairly large surgical base of patients to help me in understanding the treatment of posterolateral knee injuries. In closely following these patients, I found that the sling-type procedures that I had been taught,[18] or attempts at a primary repair in chronic injuries, frequently resulted in patients having recurrent instability. I felt that this was unacceptable, although many of my colleagues who discussed these issues with me felt it was inevitable for these injury patterns to stretch out because of the differences in bony anatomy and the normal increased physiologic laxity compared with the medial compartment of the knee. As I had found that the literature and history of primary repairs of chronic anterior and PCL injuries were similar in the results to what I was finding clinically, I sought to develop a reconstructive technique to treat posterolateral knee injuries. As my studies and those of others had indicated that the popliteus tendon, popliteofibular ligament, and the fibular collateral ligament were the main structures that needed to be reconstructed with these injury patterns, I sought to develop a reconstructive procedure for these three main structures.

My first attempt at a reconstructive procedure for the posterolateral corner of the knee was to use a split an Achilles tendon allograft with one bone plug anchored in the femur. I placed the bone plug in the femur midway between the attachment points of the fibular collateral ligament and the popliteus tendon. The more posterior strand of this split Achilles tendon allograft was then run through a tunnel in the fibula through the attachment site of the fibular collateral ligament and it exited along the posteromedial aspect of the fibular styloid at the attachment site of the popliteofibular ligament. The second strand's reconstructive graft passed through the popliteal hiatus, along the intraarticular course of the popliteus tendon, and then was sutured to the fibular collateral ligament strand. At time zero, this reconstruction helped very well to eliminate varus instability and posterolateral rotation of the tibia on the femur. I performed this reconstructive technique in 54 patients over the course of 2 years. Overall, I found that these patients were doing better than those who had undergone a primary repair with recess type procedures, bone block advancement procedures, or other primary repair type techniques.[13,17–22,24–26,35] However, at about the same point in time, reviewing the ACL and PCL literature led me to believe that placing one bone block to reconstruct both these structures was nothing more than a less modified sling procedure and was relatively nonanatomic. At the same point in time, we were also completing our quantitative anatomy study on the attachment sites of the fibular collateral ligament, popliteus tendon, and popliteofibular ligament.[36] Once I recognized that the distance between the two femoral attachment sites averaged 18.5 mm, I felt that two separate tunnels would need to be drilled at the attachment sites of both the fibular collateral ligament and the popliteus tendon on the femur to allow for a more anatomic reconstructive technique. It would appear that with the large distance between these two attachment sites, a single graft that is used to reconstruct the popliteus complex and the fibular collateral ligament, placed centrally between these femoral attachments, would be at a higher risk of stretching out and failing since it would not reproduce the normal anatomy.

Due to my frequent travels and interaction with colleagues where we describe these issues, I then further developed a relationship with the University

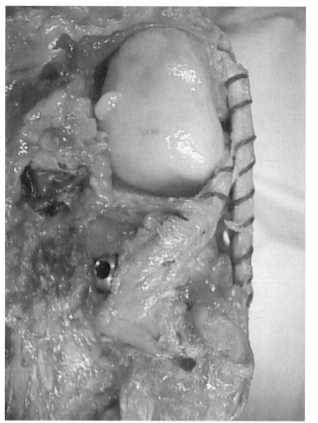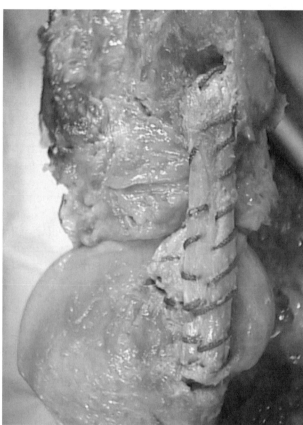

Figure 7–20   Posterior **(A)** and lateral **(B)** views of split Achilles posterolateral reconstruction with bone block in tibia (pilot study, right knee).

of Oslo where we agreed to have faculty exchanges to perform collaborative research projects. We agreed that our first project would be to work on redeveloping an anatomic posterolateral reconstructive technique and to perform a thorough biomechanical analysis on its ability to reproduce normal mechanics prior to attempting any surgical implants in patients.

Our first attempt at this type of reconstructive technique used a split Achilles tendon allograft that was placed into the posteromedial aspect of the tibia at the musculotendinous junction of the popliteus (**Fig. 7–20**). One of the split Achilles tendon arms then coursed proximally into the joint intraarticularly and was placed into a tunnel drilled at the anatomic attachment site of the popliteus tendon at the top of the popliteal sulcus. This portion of the graft reconstructed the popliteus tendon. The second portion of the split Achilles tendon allograft was placed through a drill hole in the fibula, which entered and exited at the attachment sites of the popliteofibular ligament and the fibular collateral ligament. This split graft was then passed through this fibular tunnel and placed under the anterior arm of the long head of the biceps femoris and the superficial layer of the iliotibial band to enter a femoral tunnel that was placed at the fibular collateral ligament anatomic attachment site.

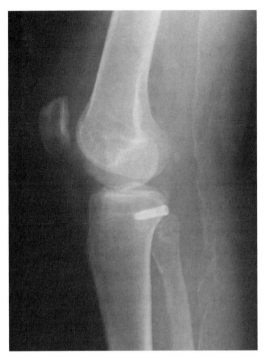

Figure 7–21   Lateral radiograph, left knee, demonstrating placement of the bone plug for a split Achilles tendon graft for the technique placing one bone plug in the tibia.

This reconstructive technique worked beautifully in the laboratory and our initial evaluation of it seemed to show that it reproduced very well the course of these structures and their biomechanical characteristics. In fact, my early enthusiasm with this analysis led me to perform six of these procedures in patients, as I felt I had proven to myself it was a better reconstructive technique to utilize than the one femoral bone block Achilles tendon split graft reconstructive procedure.

However, although this procedure worked very well in the laboratory, there were many technical issues that we encountered in patients. First, in spite of my extensive dissection history, and what I felt was a fairly good knowledge of where to put the bone block on the tibia **(Fig. 7–21)**, I found that I could not reproducibly place this bone block in the desired tibial position. In many instances, the tibial tunnel was 1 to 2 cm more distal down the tibia than it should have been, which made the reconstruction of the popliteofibular ligament and popliteus tendon a sling-type procedure. In addition, I found it very difficult to pass an eyelet-tipped guide pin consistently through the desired location over the posterolateral tibia to exit anteromedial on the tibia so the passing sutures for the bone plug will be pulled into place, after the tunnel was reamed. The other technical issue that I encountered was in applying the correct tension to each individual arm of the reconstructive graft in the femoral tunnels. It was very difficult to determine the length of the reconstructive grafts and to then drill appropriately sized tunnels to make sure that these lengths were not too short to obtain a good fixation, or to have the grafts too long so as not be able to tighten them up within the femoral tunnels and then have to shorten the ends and replace the whip stitch on the end of the graft. I found this to be very tedious and tiring once these grafts had been placed in patients. I then went back and reviewed these patients and while I felt that they were doing well clinically in the initial follow-up, I also felt that these technical issues would not allow a reconstructive technique to be adapted by surgeons who do not have the same familiarity with surgical approaches and anatomy of the posterolateral corner of the knee. I discussed this issue with Lars Engebretsen and Steinar Johansen, and came up with our current reconstructive graft procedure.[37,38] It uses a large portion of the approach and tunnel placement of many of my previous "prototype" reconstructive procedures, but we also found it to be a reproducible technique, which in our research laboratory led to excellent surgical results. We then performed this new reconstructive procedure in a series of cadaveric knees, verifying its biomechanical ability to restore the normal force and stability patterns for posterolateral knee structures **(Fig. 7–22)**. Following these biomechanical cutting and buckle transducer studies, the three of us operated on fresh whole human cadavers at the University of Oslo anatomy laboratory to assess our ability to perform this reconstruction in a reproducible manner. We were able to perform this procedure reproducibly and noted no complications with bone tunnel placement, bone tunnel fracturing, tunnel malposition, or in passing the reconstructive grafts. We then felt comfortable to proceed with performing this anatomic reconstructive procedure in patients.

The following section reviews this reconstruction procedure. I provide tips and pearls based on our collective experience of over 100 anatomic posterolateral reconstructions to date. Currently, both of our research centers have an ongoing prospective outcome study on this procedure.

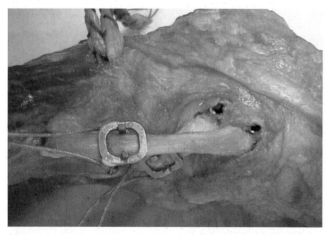

Figure 7–22 Lateral view, left knee of buckle transducers on the fibular collateral ligament and popliteus tendon limbs of the posterolateral reconstruction technique.

◆ Surgical Treatment of Chronic Posterolateral Knee Injuries

The treatment algorithms for grade 3 chronic posterolateral corner knee injuries are different from those for acute posterolateral knee injuries. For these chronic injuries, it is important to assess a patient's knee alignment prior to any consideration of a soft tissue reconstruction procedure because it has been well demonstrated that a failure to correct genu varus alignment frequently results in stretching out of the operative repair or reconstructive technique.[1,9,39] The varus alignment and the resultant thrusting and lateral compartment gapping with foot strike place excessive tension on the repaired or reconstructed lateral structures, which can lead to stretching out of these posterolateral knee grafts over time. Therefore, it is important to correct any amount of genu varus alignment of the lower extremity prior to any soft tissue reconstructions of the posterolateral corner of the knee to minimize the chance that the soft tissue reconstructions would stretch out.

A useful tool that I have found in screening patients who have some varus alignment, but in whom it is difficult to determine whether they have a symptomatic posterolateral corner injury or a variant of increased native laxity to the posterolateral corner structures, is a medial compartment unloader brace that helps determine which patients may benefit from a proximal tibial osteotomy (**Fig. 7–23**). Patients who utilize the unloader brace and have improvement of their instability pattern, with or without an alleviation of any potential associated medial compartment knee pain, have been found to have a good chance of having their instability improved with a proximal tibial osteotomy.

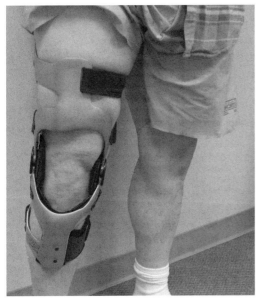

Figure 7–23   A patient wearing a medial compartment unloader brace for posterolateral knee instability (right knee).

We have found through our biomechanical testing that a proximal tibial opening wedge osteotomy results in a significant increase in both the varus and external rotation stability to a knee that has grade 3 posterolateral corner injury (see Chapter 6). In light of this, we have recommended that a proximal tibial opening wedge osteotomy be performed rather than a closing wedge proximal tibial osteotomy to take advantage of this increased tightness of these structures, which contributes to an improved overall stability for these posterolateral corner injuries.

Technique of Proximal Tibial Opening Wedge Osteotomy for Genu Varus and Chronic Posterolateral Instability

As part of the preoperative planning for chronic posterolateral knee injuries, a long leg standing hip-to-ankle anteroposterior (AP) radiograph is obtained to determine where the mechanical axis falls through the knee. For those patients who have a mechanical axis that falls medial to the tip of the medial tibial spine, we recommend a proximal tibial opening wedge osteotomy to address this varus alignment to minimize the chance of the reconstruction grafts from stretching out. It is recommended that patients who have varus alignment have this corrected first. I have learned that some patients in whom the weight-bearing axis was falling to the medial aspect of the downslope of the medial tibial spine, and who did not have a severe varus alignment that needed correction, subsequently went on to have stretching out of the reconstructive grafts over time when I did not perform an osteotomy. Thus I have followed the recommendations of my European colleagues to perform a proximal tibial opening wedge osteotomy on all patients who have any amount of varus malalignment.

In addition to correction of the coronal plane malalignment, it is important to assess sagittal plane correction for these patients. For patients who may have a concurrent ACL instability, it is recommended to tilt the sagittal slope anteriorly to address this laxity pattern (**Fig. 7–24**). In patients who have a concurrent PCL tear, combined with a chronic posterolateral knee injury, it is recommended to increase the posterior slope of the tibia. Likewise, in those patients who have a grade 3 posterolateral corner injury combined with genu recurvatum, with no other major ligament injuries seen in the knee, it is recommended to correct both the coronal plane and the sagittal plane alignment by increasing the sagittal slope of the tibia posteriorly. Patients with an isolated grade 3 posterolateral corner injury, with either no associated cruciate ligament injury or genu recurvatum, undergo a pure valgus opening, possibly with just a slight amount of increased posterior slope (because of the small primary role of the posterolateral structures in preventing posterior translation of the tibia on the femur near extension),[40–43] of their proximal tibia.

In most patients, we perform a proximal tibial opening wedge osteotomy acutely with allograft bone graft supplementation. However, in smokers or in patients whose osteopenic tibial bone stock proximally is too questionable to allow for early range of motion or in whom we are concerned about healing due to a large amount of varus malalignment, a proximal tibial distraction osteotomy may be performed.

For an acute proximal tibial wedge osteotomy, the standard surgical incision is made vertically on the tibia midway between the tibial tubercle and the

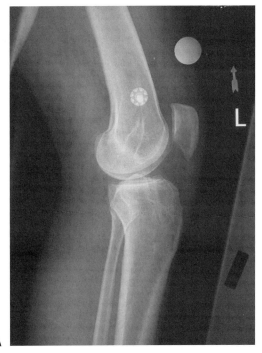
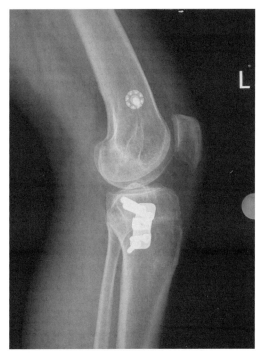

A

B

Figure 7–24 Preoperative **(A)** and postoperative **(B)** proximal tibial osteotomy radiographs. These demonstrate the sagittal plane difference in improved neutral positioning of the knee in an anterior cruciate ligament deficient knee with a concurrent posterolateral corner injury after an osteotomy that decreased the tibial slope (lateral view, left knee).

posterior border of the tibia. The incision is carried down from just distal to the joint line to just distal to the midportion of the tibial tubercle along this location. If previous incisions have been made in this region, they should be used again if possible to minimize the chance of wound breakdown between incisions.

It is recommended that the knee incision be performed directly down to bone and then a subperiosteal dissection performed. I have found that by directly incising down to bone, there is minimal skin flap formation in this location. This is important because if one dissects down slowly layer by layer, there may be more soft tissue trauma created, and I have found that in my earlier cases, or in consultation with colleagues who perform only a few of these cases a year, there is a higher likelihood that these incisions will drain when they are not carried down directly to bone. A subperiosteal dissection is performed anteriorly under the deep infrapatella bursa and patellar tendon just proximal to the tibial tubercle.[44] The dissection is performed with a small periosteal elevator and is dissected over to the level of Gerdy's tubercle. A small z-retractor is then placed into this location to allow for identification of where to make the proximal tibial anterior cut. It is important in this location to use a flat periosteal elevator when performing the subperiosteal dissection because there is a high likelihood of entering the metaphyseal bone of the proximal tibia with a curved elevator here. When this happens, it is more difficult to insert the distraction devices to open up the medial cortex without having further bone fragmentation occur.

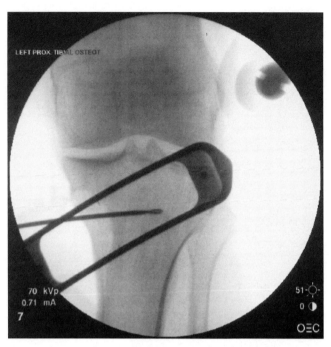

Figure 7–25 Fluoroscopic anteroposterior (AP) view of guide pin in place for the proximal tibial osteotomy demonstrating that it is parallel to the joint line (left knee).

The posterior dissection is performed in a similar fashion. A small straight elevator is used to perform a subperiosteal dissection under the tibial collateral ligament, and then a curved periosteal elevator is used to dissect the popliteus musculature off the proximal tibia posteriorly. It is important at this location to dissect across the posterior aspect of the tibia right up against the tibia itself. One should audibly hear the elevator scraping the tibia during this part of the approach. A radiolucent retractor can then be placed posteriorly to allow for visualization intraoperatively. Fluoroscopic imaging is now utilized to place two parallel guidewires along the joint line just distal to the flare of the proximal medial tibia **(Fig. 7–25)**. The slope of these guidewires is placed to attempt to duplicate the desired sagittal slope of the proximal tibia once the osteotomy cut is completed. The AP and lateral fluoroscopic planes are frequently visualized. Once the two guidewires are in the desired position, an oscillating saw performs the osteotomy, with osteotomes used to complete the cut anteriorly and posteriorly **(Fig. 7–26)**. The radiolucent retractor is very useful in this circumstance to allow for protection of the posterior neurovascular bundle and to efficiently and confidently perform the osteotomy along this posterior location **(Fig. 7–27)**. An attempt is made to preserve the lateral-most 1 cm of the tibia upon which the osteotomy is hinged.

Once it has been confirmed via lateral fluoroscopy that the anterior and posterior cortices of the tibia have been cut, a spreader device is then placed into the osteotomy to allow for a slow opening distraction to occur. It is important to do this slowly, to allow for stress relaxation of the lateral tibial cortical bone to prevent cracking of the lateral cortex or an intraarticular extension

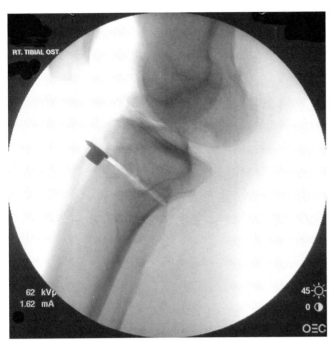

Figure 7–26 Lateral fluoroscopic view showing the osteotome completing the anterior cortex cut for a proximal tibial opening wedge osteotomy (right knee).

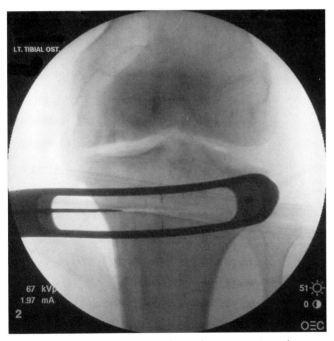

Figure 7–27 Retractor in place demonstrating the protection of the posterior structures while performing a proximal tibial opening wedge osteotomy (left knee).

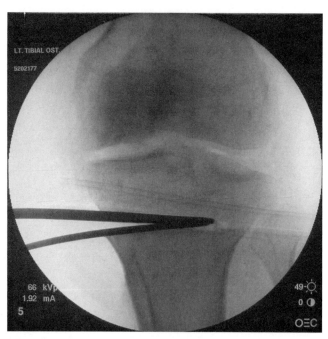

Figure 7–28   Opening wedge spreader device in place for a proximal tibial opening wedge osteotomy (fluoroscopic view, left knee).

(Fig. 7–28). In some of the earlier procedures that I performed with sports medicine fellows, we found that overzealousness and an attempt to perform this distraction rather quickly can lead to cracking of the lateral cortex, which can result in instability of the junction between the osteotomy sites, or intraarticular fractures. For this reason, I try to go very slowly to make sure that the lateral cortex remains intact. If it does not, I do not hesitate to make an incision over Gerdy's tubercle and to place a bone staple to provide stability to the lateral cortex of the osteotomy site prior to placing the plate medially.

Once the osteotomy has been opened to the calculated amount, the spreader device is then removed and the plate is inserted. In those circumstances where I wish to decrease the slope of the proximal tibia, the angled (sloped) plate is placed as far posteriorly as possible along the proximal tibia. In those cases in which I want to increase the posterior slope of the tibia, the plate is placed along the anteromedial aspect of the tibia. When angled plates are used, the higher portion of the angled plate is placed at the apex of the desired change in slope angulation. The screws for the higher portion of the plate are then secured proximally and distally. The knee is then slowly extended and the tibial slope will be changed as the proximal tibia closes down over the narrower portion of the plate. Standard screw fixation is then completed for the remaining plate holes.

After plate fixation is achieved, bone graft is then placed into the osteotomy site. I prefer to use commercially prepared allograft bone in the osteotomy site to try to pack as much bone in as possible and to minimize the morbidity associated

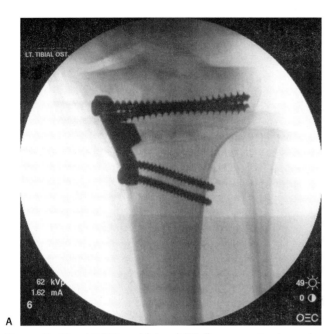
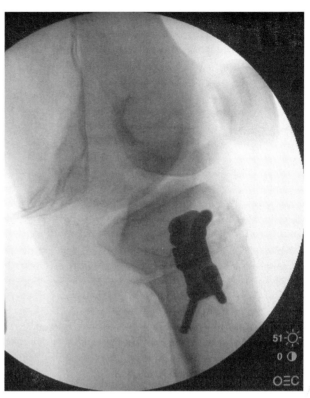

Figure 7–29   AP **(A)** and lateral **(B)** fluoroscopic views demonstrating bone graft in place after a proximal tibial opening wedge osteotomy (left knee).

with iliac crest bone graft harvesting (**Fig. 7–29**). I have minimally used bone morphogenic protein to speed up bone healing at this point in the procedure.

As a final step, AP and lateral fluoroscopic imaging is utilized to check to make sure that there is complete packing of the opening wedge osteotomy site with allograft bone graft, as well as to verify that there is no protrusion of the bone graft either anteriorly or posteriorly from the osteotomy site. If any graft protrusion is noted, periosteal elevators are used to either pack down the knee graft into the osteotomy site or to remove the excess bone graft at this time.

Copious irrigation with normal saline is performed over the osteotomy site to remove any bone debris from the saw or excess allograft bone graft prior to closure. I believe it is very important to remove this debris, or any excess allograft, from the site to minimize the chance of drainage postoperatively. The periosteum is closed over the plate, followed by closure of the subcutaneous tissues, and a subcuticular suturing of the skin is performed.

Our standard postoperative rehabilitation protocol for these patients is to allow them immediate full range of motion as tolerated, with a goal of obtaining at least 90 degrees of knee flexion by 2 weeks postoperatively. Patients are allowed to remove their immobilizers four times daily to work on range of motion. They are kept non–weight-bearing for the initial 8 weeks postoperatively. During this time, they perform quadriceps sets and straight leg raises several times daily in the immobilizer only. I recommend that patients remain in their immobilizers at all times, except when performing range-of-motion exercises, as an insurance against injuring themselves in a fall.

Plain AP and lateral radiographs are obtained on these knees at 2, 8, and 12 weeks postoperatively. The radiographs obtained at 2 weeks are obtained to verify the position of the bone graft and hardware to supplement the fluoroscopic imaging views obtained intraoperatively. The radiographs obtained at 8 weeks are used to compare with the 2-week radiographs to verify that there is still an intact lateral cortex and that there is starting to be evidence of early consolidation of the trabecular bone on the lateral aspect of the osteotomy. If this is present, patients are then allowed to progressively increase their weight bearing by 25% of their body weight per week until they are fully weight bearing 3 months postoperatively. Repeat AP and lateral radiographs of the knee are once again obtained at that time. If there is evidence of continued consolidation of the osteotomy site with healing, as well as no evidence of any subsidence of the osteotomy or bending of the screws, the patients are then allowed to wean themselves off the crutches as tolerated and when they can walk without a limp. They are then put on a progressive strengthening program. They are allowed to participate in a low-impact exercise program and to use an exercise bike, to swim, to do leg presses to a maximum of 70 degrees of knee flexion, and to do a general ambulation program.

Patients return to the clinic at 6 months postoperatively, at which time we obtain repeat AP and lateral radiographs of their knee as well as a long leg alignment radiograph to verify the results of the corrective coronal plane osteotomy. We also review the patients' functional status to determine if a second-stage soft tissue reconstruction is needed to address the overall instability. Some patients feel that they have enough stability created by the osteotomy itself and that they do not need a second-stage reconstruction. Several of my European colleagues believe that half of patients who have had a proximal tibial opening wedge osteotomy do not need a second-stage posterolateral corner reconstruction. In our prospective study to date, which is still ongoing, it appears that the number of patients who do need a second-stage posterolateral corner reconstruction after a proximal tibial opening wedge osteotomy is higher than 50%, but I have noted that there are several patients who are quite satisfied with the result of the osteotomy and feel that they do not need a second-stage reconstructive procedure. Therefore, I always tell my patients preoperatively that we need to have them properly rehabilitated after the osteotomy and that they need to tell me if they are having functional limitations after the osteotomy to determine if they need a second-stage soft tissue reconstruction once the osteotomy has healed completely.

In those patients who do need a second-stage soft tissue reconstruction of their posterolateral structures, possibly combined with a concurrent cruciate ligament reconstruction, it is important to make sure that the osteotomy site is completely healed prior to doing the reconstruction (**Fig. 7–30**). This is especially important for patients who need a concurrent ACL or PCL reconstruction procedure because the bone tunnels will pass through the osteotomy site on the medial aspect of the knee, which tends to consolidate later than the lateral aspect. Our average time frame to proceed with a second-stage soft tissue reconstruction after these proximal tibial opening wedge osteotomies is approximately 8 to 9 months postoperatively.

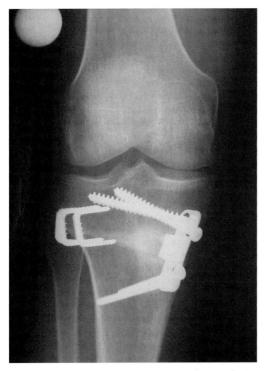

Figure 7–30 Postoperative AP radiograph 6 months after a proximal tibial opening wedge osteotomy demonstrating healing when the patient was ready for a second-stage posterolateral corner reconstructive surgery (right knee, staples due to lateral cortex fracture while removing failed PCL reconstruction tibial screw).

I have not found that hardware removal and subsequent potential concurrent cruciate ligament reconstruction significantly affect operative time during a second-stage soft tissue reconstructive procedure. The only time where I have found any technical issues related to this is when the plate removal location is at the same location as an ACL reconstruction graft tibial tunnel. In these instances, I think it is important to position the tibial guide pin for an ACL reconstruction tibial tunnel to avoid this location and to prevent an excessively large tibial tunnel aperture opening.

Surgical Treatment for Grade III Chronic Posterolateral Knee Injuries with Normal or Corrected Lower Extremity Alignment

Although there may be instances where a primary repair of grade 3 posterolateral corner chronic injuries may be possible, in the majority of circumstances it is usually not possible due to scar tissue formation, retraction of torn structures, and the fact that these previously injured structures tend to stretch out once they are repaired. Thus I have advocated that a reconstructive procedure be performed, which anatomically restores the anatomy of the course and quantitative attachment sites of the three main static stabilizers of the posterolateral corner of the knee[38]: the fibular collateral ligament, popliteus tendon, and popliteofibular ligament. Previous techniques to reconstruct the posterolateral corner structures have included fibular collateral ligament reconstructions, femoral bone block advancements of the attachment sites of the posterolateral corner structures, biceps femoris tenodesis, popliteus tendon, and popliteofibular ligament reconstruction using split patellar tendon grafts; popliteus tendon recess procedures; and central slip iliotibial band or biceps femoris grafts.[13,15,17–22,24,25,35] The purpose of these operative techniques is to restore varus and external rotatory static stability to knees that exhibit significant and symptomatic posterolateral rotatory instability. However, although the surgical techniques may provide varying degrees of stability to knees with these injuries, I believe that a large portion of these procedures are sling procedures that do not anatomically reconstruct the main structures of the posterolateral corner of the knee or rely on a primary repair of injured structures that tend to stretch out over time.

We look at the patient's history to determine what type of reconstructive procedures should be performed for the posterolateral corner of the knee. It took many years before it became evident that quantitative, anatomic, and biomechanical studies of the native ACL and PCL were crucial in helping to determine appropriate graft locations and to develop proper cruciate ligament reconstructive techniques.[29,34] These studies have shown that those grafts which reconstruct the normal anatomy of the cruciate ligaments provide the best restoration of normal knee function. It has been well demonstrated that for both the ACL and the PCL, anatomic reconstructions result in the best outcome in reducing abnormal joint motion and improving patient overall function.

Anatomic Posterolateral Reconstruction Technique

Preoperative planning for proper performance of a posterolateral corner reconstruction procedure is essential. I do not use a leg holder and prefer to place a sandbag taped at the foot of the bed to allow for about 70-degree knee flexion to provide access to the posterolateral corner of the knee. In addition, I very commonly place a sandbag under the patient's hip so that the knee will balance at 70 degrees intraoperatively. Then the assistants can retract tissues rather than have to hold the knee in position.

The posterolateral corner reconstruction technique utilizes standard cruciate ligament reconstruction instruments. Cannulated guides from cruciate ligament reconstruction systems are utilized for positioning of the guide pins during the tunnel placement. Islet-tipped passing pins are also utilized to pass sutures and to ream over these pins when tunnels are placed. Cannulated metal and bioabsorbable screws are used to provide fixation of the grafts, as well as small bone staples to provide secure graft backup fixation. The Achilles tendon graft utilized for the procedure should be at least 23 cm long to ensure that it can pass through the varying courses of the posterolateral corner reconstructive technique (**Tables 7–1** and **7–2**).

Surgical Approach for the Posterolateral Corner Reconstruction Procedure

The skin incision for the posterolateral corner reconstruction is the same as for an acute repair of the posterolateral corner. Issues with the placement of the skin incision are usually less important than in the acute situation and one does

Table 7–1 Instrumentation and Setup for Posterolateral Reconstructions

Instrumentation Needs	Setup Needs
A transtibial or transfemoral ACL/PCL guide system	No leg holder
Beath passing pins with eyelets	Sandbag taped to bed to allow for 70 degrees of knee flexion
Cannulated 7- and 9-mm reamers	Bump under hip to allow for neutral position of knee during positioning
Cannulated 7- and 9-mm (bioabsorbable) interference screws	Various retractors
A soft tissue staple fixation system	Achilles tendon allograft ≥23 cm long (with calcaneous bone plug)
Atsen tipped hemostat for peroneal nerve neurolysis/fine dissection	

not have to worry about degloving issues or significant preincision hematomas. However, I try to leave at least a 6- to 7-cm skin bridge between the anterior incision for a cruciate ligament reconstruction procedure and the posterolateral corner surgical approach.

The skin incision is made using a lateral hockey-stick incision unless previous skin incisions need to be incorporated. The incision is centered over Gerdy's tubercle and extends proximally along the posterior border of the iliotibial band and anteriorly over the anterior compartment of the leg. The incision is carried down to the superficial layer of the iliotibial band and the fascia covering the anterior compartment of the leg. A posteriorly based skin flap is then developed by meticulously dissecting along this layer until one reaches the long head of the biceps femoris. Once I get to this location, I perform a common peroneal nerve neurolysis to remove it from any resultant scar tissue, as well as to allow the nerve to be retracted away it from the surgical field.

Table 7–2 Surgical Pearls of the Posterolateral Reconstruction

I	A 1-cm horizontal incision through the anterior arm of the long biceps facilitates identification of the fibular collateral ligament.
II	A suture placed into the fibular collateral ligament, through the biceps bursa, facilitates identification of its course and potentially its femoral attachment site.
III	Placement of the transfemoral eyelet pins should aim through the anatomic attachment sites of the popliteus tendon and fibular collateral ligament laterally to slightly proximal and anterior to the adductor tubercle on the anteromedial aspect of the knee.
IV	The entry site anteriorly for the tibial reconstructive tunnel should be just distal and medial to Gerdy's tubercle along its flat spot; lateral to this, the tibia downslopes at the anterior compartment and it is difficult to place in a proper tunnel and obtain fixation.
V	The initial part of the surgical procedure may be performed without a tourniquet; the initial surgical approach, identification of the fibular collateral ligament through the biceps bursa, the common peroneal nerve neurolysis, and identification and reaming of the fibular head and tibial tunnels may be done with minimal bleeding.

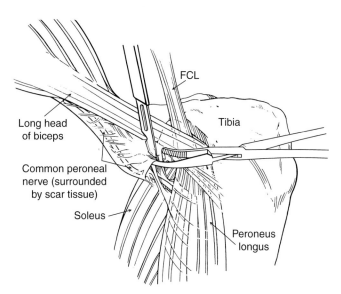

Figure 7–31 The Adson tipped hemostat holding up scar tissue away from the common peroneal nerve during a nerve decompression, while an assistant cuts the scar with a No. 15 scalpel blade (lateral view, right knee).

In the chronic situation, the common peroneal nerve can usually be identified by direct palpation. In those cases where there is a significant amount of scar tissue present, the common peroneal nerve may need to be identified proximally where it is just crossing posteriorly under the long head of the biceps tendon. In those instances where there may be significant scar in this location, the peroneal nerve can usually be palpated approximately 2 cm distal to the lateral aspect of the fibular head. A small incision through the peroneus longus fascia in this location and then gentle dissection posterior to the musculature can usually identify the nerve here if it is difficult to find it more proximally along its course. I prefer to use an Adsen tipped hemostat to allow me to gently dissect around the nerve while an assistant uses a No. 15 surgical blade to gently release the scar tissue planes, which I hold up between the points of the hemostat, which encompass the nerve at this location (**Fig. 7–31**). Once the nerve has been freed from the scar tissue in this location, a small Penrose drain is then placed around it to allow for gentle retraction away from the surgical fields intraoperatively. Once the common peroneal nerve has been retracted away from the surgical field, one can bluntly dissect in the interval between the lateral gastrocnemius and the soleus muscles to gain access to the popliteofibular ligament attachment on the posteromedial aspect of the fibular head and styloid as well as to palpate medially along the proximal posterior tibia to identify the PCL attachment facet on the tibia.

Identification of the Fibular Collateral Ligament and Fibular Attachment Site, and Fibular Tunnel Placement   The next phase in the posterolateral corner reconstruction procedure is to identify the fibular collateral ligament attachment site on the fibula. In a similar fashion to what is done in acute injuries, a small horizontal incision is made through the anterior arm of the long head of the biceps femoris, about 1 cm proximal to where it attaches on the lateral aspect of the fibular head. Once one incises through the biceps bursa in this location, the distal aspect of the fibular collateral ligament, or a remnant of the ligament, can almost always be found deep to it. A traction stitch can be placed into the ligament to assist in defining its proximal attachment site on the femur (**Fig. 7–7**). In the majority of these chronic injuries, I have found that the fibular collateral ligament is stretched out, rather than torn intrasubstance, and tugging on the fibular collateral ligament distally facilitates finding its femoral attachment site. There have been cases where up to 3 cm of increased lateral compartment opening has been found on varus stress radiographs and an intact, but very attenuated, fibular collateral ligament is present.

Once this retraction stitch has been placed into the fibular collateral ligament, attention is turned toward identification of the exact attachment site of the fibular collateral ligament on the lateral aspect of the fibula head. The anterior arm of the biceps femoris is carefully dissected off its anterior and distal fibular head attachment sites to identify the outline of the lateral aspect of the fibular head. The more proximal biceps attachment site, including the direct arm of long head of the biceps femoris, is left intact at its attachment site on the fibular head and styloid. It is important to recognize where the common peroneal nerve is during this portion of the dissection, so that the dissection is not performed any further distally than is necessary to minimize irritation of the common peroneal nerve, and so that the nerve is not injured. The fibular head in this location is shaped like a champagne glass and there is a rapid drop-off to the fibular shaft. One needs to stay directly against bone and to avoid distal dissection of the anterior arm of the long biceps to prevent injury to the common peroneal nerve because it is only 1 to 2 cm distal to this location. In most instances, there is at least a portion of the fibular collateral ligament attachment site left on the lateral aspect of the fibular head. In our anatomic studies, we have found that the fibular collateral ligament attaches at an average of 38% from anterior to posterior along the lateral aspect of the fibular head.[36] This number can be utilized to help find the fibular attachment site when it may have been damaged previously and no remnant is able to be visualized. Once I identify the exact anatomic site of the fibular collateral ligament on the fibula, which is where I will drill the guide pin, I use a small curved elevator to identify the posteromedial downslope of the fibular styloid. This is the location where the popliteofibular ligament will attach. Once I have outlined this area, I insert a cannulated cruciate ligament guide, which enables the guide pin to enter the fibular head at the fibular collateral ligament attachment site and to exit along the posteromedial aspect of the fibular head and styloid (**Fig. 7–32**). A 7-mm cannulated reamer is then reamed over this guide pin to allow for creation of the fibular tunnel. It is important either to palpate directly over the posteromedial fibula or to use a posterior retractor to make sure that the guide pin does not overpenetrate at that location and injure the neurovascular structures. The usual length of the fibular tunnel is 25 to 30 mm. When one is learning how to ream these tunnels, I would suggest leaving only about 25 to 30 mm of guide pin between the cannulated guide and the power chuck to make sure the guide pin does not overpenetrate posteriorly because this is the usual length of the fibular tunnel.

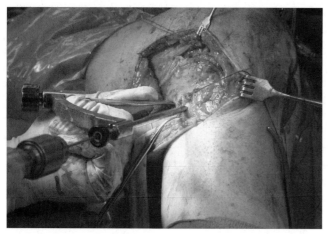

Figure 7–32 The fibular head tunnel guide pin in place (lateral view, right knee, traction stitch in remaining FCL substance).

When drilling this tunnel, make sure that it has adequate bone stock, and verify that you are reproducing the normal anatomic attachment sites for these structures (**Fig. 7–33**). In some instances, the tunnels may need to be placed slightly distal along the fibular shaft; make sure that the reamed tunnel does not break out proximally through either the fibular head or the styloid (**Table 7–3**). It is also important to have some type of retraction protecting the neurovascular bundle when one is both drilling and overreaming the guide pin for the tunnel. A small hand-held rasp can then be placed through the fibular tunnel to make sure that there are no sharp edges along its medial aspect and to clean out soft tissue debris after it has been reamed.

Preparation of the Tibial Tunnel for the Posterolateral Corner Reconstruction Procedure   After the fibular tunnel has been drilled, it is possible to proceed with drilling the tibial tunnel for this reconstruction procedure. The tunnel enters anteriorly on the tibia and exits posteriorly at the popliteus musculotendinous junction. There are some important anatomic landmarks to recognize when drilling this tunnel. First, the anterior entry site should be placed slightly distal and medial to Gerdy's tubercle. In this location, which is just lateral to the deep infrapatellar bursa and the patellar tendon itself, there is a flat space on the proximal tibia, which allows one to drill a tunnel and have good bone stock surrounding it. I have found that if one moves slightly lateral to this space that the champagne glass–shaped lateral curvature of the anterior compartment results in a much shorter bone tunnel that sometimes can be close to the proximal tibiofibular joint. It also makes fixation with a soft tissue staple more difficult. Therefore, the best fixation does appear to be when one drills this tunnel slightly distal and medial to Gerdy's tubercle, where there is a flat spot to obtain better purchase for the graft's tibial fixation later in the case.

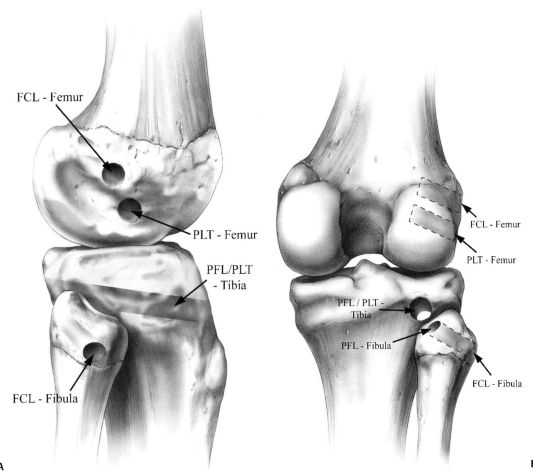

A

B

Figure 7–33 Posterolateral reconstruction tunnel lateral **(A)** and posterior **(B)** views (FCL, fibular collateral ligament; PLT, popliteus tendon; PFL, popliteofibular ligament). (From LaPrade RF, Johansen S, Wentorf FA, Engebretsen L, Esterberg JL, Tso A. An analysis of an anatomic posterolateral knee reconstruction: an *in vitro* biomechanical study and development of a surgical technique. Am J Sports Med 2004;32: 1405–1414, with permission.)

Table 7–3   Pitfalls in the Posterolateral Corner Reconstructive Procedure

I	Do not place the fibular head tunnel too proximal. It may not preserve a good cortical rim of bone at the superior aspect of the fibular tunnel.
II	Drilling the tibial tunnel too distal at its exit site on the posterolateral tibia could result in a horizontal popliteofibular ligament graft. The tibial tunnel posteriorly should exit 8 to 10 mm proximal from the exit site of the fibular head tunnel. Therefore, the fibular head tunnel should be reamed first, to serve as a reference guide, prior to drilling the tibial tunnel.
III	Placing the transfemoral eyelet pins too parallel to the joint may result in the passing sutures going through the intercondylar notch or the guide pins hitting a posterior cruciate ligament femoral tunnel.
IV	Not tubularizing the reconstructive grafts accurately at their ends may result in them bunching up when attempting to pass them through the fibula, or tibial, tunnels.

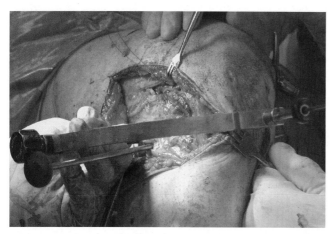

Figure 7–34 The tibial guide pin in place, the blunt obturator placed through the fibular head tunnel to serve as a reference guide, and drilling the tibial guide pin from anterior to posterior (lateral view, right knee).

In terms of the posterior landmarks for the tibial tunnel, it is important to recognize that we are trying to reproduce the normal course of the popliteus tendon and the popliteofibular ligament. The location where we drill the tunnel posteriorly is at the musculotendinous junction of the popliteus complex. At this location, there is a small, palpable sulcus on the posterolateral aspect of the tibia that can be identified once an elevator is used to prepare this area for drilling the tunnel.[14,45] In addition, one can help to identify this location by placing in a blunt obturator from an arthroscope into the fibular tunnel. The tibial tunnel should exit the posterior aspect of the tibia approximately 1 cm proximal to the exit point of the fibular tunnel (which can then be palpated via the blunt obturator placed through it)[36] **(Fig. 7–34)**.

The tibial tunnel is drilled from anterior to posterior. It is very important not to overpenetrate with the guide pin in this location. Posterior retraction is placed to protect the neurovascular bundle. If one feels that the guide pin comes out in a location that does not appear to be the musculotendonous junction, especially in those instances where the tibial tunnel is parallel in the horizontal plane to the fibular tunnel, the guide pin should be taken out and repositioned to make sure that it comes out as close as possible to its anatomic position. A 9-mm reamer is used to ream from anterior to posterior with care taken not to overpenetrate significantly when reaming through the posterior cortex. I always place a posterior retractor to make sure I am protecting the neurovascular bundle. The posterior exit site of this tibial tunnel should also be chamfered with the use of a hand-held rasp to remove any bony debris.

In almost all cases, I have not used a tourniquet until identification of the femoral attachment sites of these structures is necessary. I can usually perform the surgical approach, common peroneal nerve neurolysis, and drilling of both the fibular and tibial tunnels without having to use a tourniquet.

Identification of the Femoral Attachment Sites of the Fibular Collateral Ligament and Popliteus Tendon

To identify the attachment sites of the fibular collateral ligament and popliteus tendon on the femur, a splitting incision of the superficial layer of the iliotibial band is made. The splitting incision is in the same location as would be made for a surgical approach for an acute posterolateral corner repair. The incision is centered along the posterior aspect of the iliotibial band, approximately 1 to 2 cm proximal to its posterior border, and performed down to Gerdy's tubercle. The incision ideally should cross the joint line directly over the popliteal sulcus on the femur. It is important during this portion of the surgical approach not to cut too deeply because this may injure the lateral capsule, fibular collateral ligament, or the lateral gastrocnemius tendon. I prefer to insert a hemostat along the entire course of the iliotibial band when we are making this incision to avoid injuries to any native structures, which may still be intact. Once the iliotibial band has been elevated anteriorly and posteriorly with the use of some type of retractors by the assistants, I turn my attention to identification of the femoral attachment sites of the popliteus tendon and fibular collateral ligament. If further cruciate or other knee ligament work is necessary, I hold the further steps of the posterolateral approach until all intraarticular work is completed so that there is not excessive fluid extravasation due to the lateral capsular incision that is necessary at this point.

The popliteus tendon attachment site is usually identified first. A knife handle placed along the shaft of the fibula will identify where the fibular collateral ligament course should be. The surgical incision is performed 1 cm anterior to this parallel imaginary line, which is drawn between the region of the lateral epicondyle and the fibular head. The meniscofemoral portion of the mid-third lateral capsular splitting incision is made first. Once one gets down to the level of the lateral meniscus, it is important to coagulate or ligate the inferior lateral genicular artery at this location. Anterior and posterior retraction of the incised capsule through this incision then facilitates identifying the popliteus tendon attachment on the femur as well as determining the status and integrity of the popliteomeniscal fascicles.

The normal attachment of the popliteus tendon is at the anterior and proximal-most fifth of the popliteal sulcus. In many instances, the native popliteus tendon is still intact in this location, although there may be a rather significant intrasubstance stretch injury with significant instability on clinical exam. It is important to take down the majority of the popliteus tendon attachment at this location to drill the tunnel in the desired position. However, I try to leave a few fibers of the popliteus tendon intact because these fibers may scar back in and restore some dynamic component to the popliteus reconstruction graft.

Once the popliteus attachment site on the femur has been identified, attention is turned to identification of the fibular collateral ligament's femoral attachment site. There are several ways that one can try to identify the anatomic location of this attachment site.

First, one can tug on the traction stitch placed through the biceps bursa, in the distal fibular collateral ligament to find its proximal course. Palpation of the course of the fibular collateral ligament can facilitate identifying the normal attachment site on the femur in most instances. This attachment site is slightly proximal and posterior to the lateral epicondyle, which can often be palpated. The fibular collateral ligament's femoral attachment site is in a small depression just slightly proximal and posterior to the lateral epicondyle.[8,36] If there is still a fairly stable attachment of the fibular collateral ligament in this location, the attachment site can be easily taken down and the desired position to drill the pin is marked in this location with a Bovie or methylene blue surgical marker.

Once the native attachment sites of the popliteus tendon and the fibular collateral ligament have been identified on the femur, the cruciate ligament cannulated guides are used to place an islet-tipped guide pin through each of these attachment sites, which exit medially on the femur. It is important to angulate these guide pins such that they exit on the anterior half of the femur, slightly proximal to the adductor tubercle region. If one has these islet pins cross parallel to the joint at this location, the passing sutures will pass through the intercondylar notch, or they may interfere with the femoral tunnel of a PCL reconstructive graft. Once the two guide pins have been placed parallel to each other, it is important to measure between the two attachment sites. The average distance between these two attachment sites is 18.5 mm and I always measure between these two to make sure that I am putting the guide pins in the correct locations[36] **(Fig. 7–35)**. This is especially important in those cases where the native ligament or tendon may have been torn off its attachment site(s) or where previous tunnels and hardware may have distorted these normal bony landmarks. It is important to verify that the guide pins, and subsequent tunnels, are placed in the native anatomic attachment sites. I find there are times when I misjudge where these tunnels need to be placed initially, and measuring the distance between these two guide pins provides a second stop-gap measure to confirm that the tunnels are placed in the desired positions. It is also important to verify that the popliteus tendon guide pin is slightly anterior to the fibular collateral ligament guide pin when the knee is in full extension prior to reaming those tunnels.

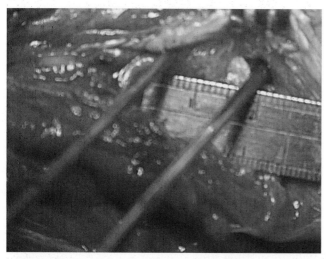

Figure 7–35   Two eyelet passing pins in place, with a ruler measuring the 18.5-mm distance between the two attachment sites (lateral view, left knee).

Preparation of the Grafts for the Posterolateral Corner Reconstruction Procedure

The grafts for the posterolateral corner reconstruction procedure are prepared either after identification of the femoral attachment sites, or after the islet tipped pins have been placed into these attachment sites. My preferred graft for this reconstruction technique is a split Achilles tendon allograft with a calcaneous bone plug. This allows me to have secure bone fixation on the femoral attachment sites with tendonous ends that can be pulled through the fibular and tibial tunnels to reconstruct these structures distally. When this type of graft may not be available due to allograft availability issues or if the patient refuses an allograft, one may use autogenous or allograft hamstring grafts as a substitute. However, the rehabilitation program postoperatively may need to be adjusted to allow for this fixation difference.

It is important to make sure that the Achilles tendon allograft that is obtained is at least 23 cm in overall length. This is the length that we have found to be necessary so that the posterolateral corner grafts can pass through the reamed tunnels.[38]

After the Achilles tendon allograft has been thawed out, the calcaneal bone plug is split in two, followed by the splitting of the tendon lengthwise, leaving good tendon substance on either side of the split **(Fig. 7–36)**. Once the calcaneal bone plug has been split lengthwise in two, 9 mm × 20 mm bone plugs are then prepared for each separate graft.

We have found that the average length of the fibular collateral ligament is about 70 mm, whereas the average length of the popliteus tendon is about 60 mm.[4,36] I choose one of the grafts to be utilized to reconstruct the fibular collateral ligament, whereas the other reconstructs the popliteus tendon at this time. The main substance of the tendon is left larger for the desired length for either the fibular collateral ligament or popliteus tendon graft (70 mm or 60 mm long, respectively). The remaining tendon graft is trimmed and tubularized distally to fit through a 7-mm tunnel. A whip stitch is placed in the ends of

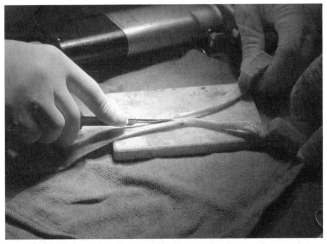

Figure 7–36 Split Achilles tendon allograft for the posterolateral corner reconstruction.

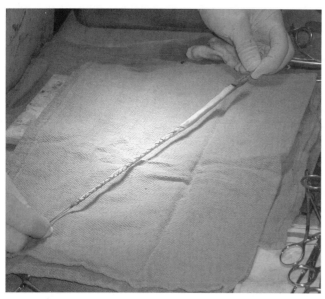

Figure 7–37 A tubularized Achilles tendon allograft for a posterolateral corner reconstruction graft.

the tendon to tubularize it to allow for passing into the tunnels (**Fig. 7–37**). It is especially important to make sure that the ends of the fibular collateral ligament graft are well tubularized to prevent any bunching up of the tissue during graft passage through the fibular bone tunnel. It can be extremely frustrating when this bunching up occurs during this late portion of the procedure, and it is very important to try to tubularize the ends to make sure that they do not bunch up when the graft is being pulled through the bony tunnel.

Posterolateral Corner Graft Fixation on the Femur

After the grafts have been prepared on the back table and their bone plugs have been appropriately sized, passing stitches are placed into the bone plugs. To make sure that the passing stitches do not break when being pulled through the femur with the eyelet-tipped guide pin, I place two No. 2 nonabsorbable sutures in each bone plug. Once this is completed, the length of the bone plugs (usually 20 to 22 mm long) is measured to determine the depth of the tunnels that will need to be reamed over the islet-tipped guide pins at the femoral attachment sites. A 9-mm reamer is used to ream to the desired depth for each of the guide pins. This depth is usually 22 to 25 mm. Once this has been completed, the tunnels need to be irrigated thoroughly to remove any bone debris so that the bone plugs will insert flush into the tunnels (**Fig. 7–38**).

Once the femoral bone tunnels have been prepared, the passing stitches in the graft bone plugs are placed into the islet-tipped pins guides and then pulled out medially on the femur. These sutures are then used to pull the bone plugs into their respective tunnels. The bone plugs should face cancellous side up with the main substance of the tendon over the distal aspect of

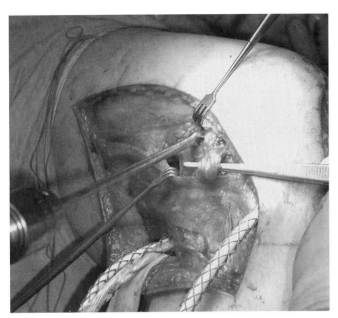

Figure 7–38   Reaming of fibular collateral ligament femoral tunnel (popliteus tendon graft under pickups, lateral view, right knee).

the tunnel **(Fig. 7–39)**. Once they have been pulled into their tunnels, they are secured in the femur with cannulated interference screws.

Placement of the cannulated guide pin for the interference screws into the femoral tunnels in this location can sometimes be problematic. I place the guide pin into a hand-held chuck with only about 4 to 5 cm sticking out the end of the chuck. This facilitates having a good handle on the guide pin, and the guide pin can then usually be easily pushed between the bone plug and the

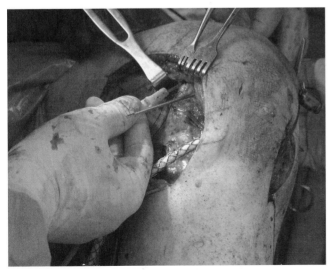

Figure 7–39   Fibular collateral ligament graft passage into the femoral tunnel. The islet-tipped pin is pulled through the femur to pull the passing sutures out medially. The sutures then pull the bone plug into the femoral tunnel (lateral view, right knee).

proximal femoral rim of the tunnel at this time. Once the guide pin is placed in the desired location, a cannulated 7-mm by 20-mm metal screw is used to allow for fixation of the bone plug in the femoral tunnel. Distal traction is then applied to the graft to verify that the bone plug fixation is secure in its femoral tunnel at this time.

Posterolateral Graft Passage and Fibular/Tibial Tunnel Fixation

Passage of the grafts is now performed. It is important to make sure that they pass along the course of the native ligaments to allow for anatomic fixation. The popliteus tendon graft is passed by placing it through the popliteal hiatus. A curved hemostat or Kocher forceps is used to follow the path of this structure and to pass the whip-stitch sutures so that they exit at the popliteus musculotendinous junction. The graft should exit posteriorly at the musculotendinous junction of the popliteus. The popliteus graft is pulled distally through this location and then attention is turned to passing the fibular collateral ligament graft.

A large curved hemostat is then placed along the native course of the fibular collateral ligament. This instrument enters through the biceps bursa and courses under the anterior arm of the long head of the biceps femoris lateral fascial attachment and under the superficial layer of the iliotibial band to enter close to the attachment site on the femur. It is important to spread the hemostat when it is in this location to make sure that there is enough room to place the allograft so it does not impinge along this course in the location. The sutures in the end of the allograft are then placed into the hemostat, and the fibular collateral ligament graft is pulled distally to exit the soft tissues close to the fibular tunnel (**Fig. 7–40**).

The graft is then passed through the fibular head and styloid from lateral to medial. A large suture with a loop tied in the end greatly helps to thread the passing sutures through the fibular tunnel. A small mosquito hemostat often helps to place this passing suture through the fibular head. Once this is performed, distal traction is performed on the graft to confirm that it is not caught proximally under the soft tissues and that it can have appropriate tension to reconstitute the normal function of the fibular collateral ligament. Once this is verified, the knee is then flexed to about 15 to 20 degrees, kept in neutral rotation, and a slight valgus force is then placed on the knee to reduce the lateral joint opening while the graft is tensioned distally. It is especially important in large patients to verify that the lateral compartment gapping is completely reduced, or there will be residual laxity to varus instability. I have noted in some morbidly obese patients that some lateral compartment gapping was present on their initial postoperative radiographs and now I am extremely careful to make sure that this does not happen again. A bioabsorbable screw is then placed in the posterior aspect of the tunnel in the fibular head along a cannulated guide pin to secure the fibular collateral ligament graft in the fibula.

I then place the leg over the side of the bed and verify that the varus instability has been eliminated. If there is any concern that possibly there is some residual laxity, I remove the screw, verify that there is no bunching up of

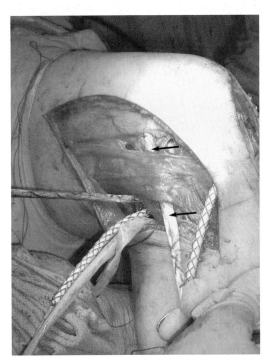

Figure 7–40 Fibular collateral ligament graft (arrows) fixation in the fibular head tunnel. The knee is placed in slight valgus and neutral rotation, at 30 degrees of knee flexion, and an assistant tugs on the graft to tighten it up. The bioabsorbable screw is then placed over a guide pin in the fibular head tunnel.

the tissue, apply further distal traction, and then reinsert a slightly larger cannulated bioabsorbable screw to obtain fixation and verify that this is stable with varus stressing at 30 degrees knee flexion. This is an extremely important point of graft evaluation, as it is the varus instability that can place significant amounts of increased stress on cruciate ligament reconstruction grafts performed concurrently and can result in functional problems with gait.

After the fibular collateral ligament graft has been fixed in the fibula, the remaining portion of this graft now reconstitutes the popliteofibular ligament. If one is able to find the musculotendinous junction of the popliteus, this portion of the popliteus tendon graft can be wrapped around the musculotendinous junction such that it will help reconstitute the dynamic function of the popliteus complex. A passing stitch is placed from anterior to posterior and then the two grafts are pulled out anteriorly simultaneously. I most commonly use a small Gore smoother (Gore Inc., Flagstaff, AZ) to facilitate graft passage in this location. It is important to cycle these grafts individually while applying distal traction to make sure there is no bunching up of the soft tissues posteriorly or any bunching up within the tibial tunnel. These two grafts now constitute the popliteus tendon and the popliteofibular ligament. Once the grafts have been pulled out anteriorly on the tibia and have been cycled and appear to reduce the abnormal posterolateral rotation present, the grafts are fixed on the tibia with a 9-mm cannulated bioabsorbable screw (**Fig. 7–41**). The knee should be in neutral rotation, at 60 degrees of knee flexion, and with distal traction on both grafts to

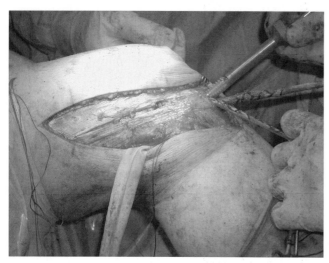

Figure 7–41   Fixation of popliteus and popliteofibular bone plugs on tibia (right knee, distal traction applied to grafts separately).

achieve fixation. I try not to internally rotate the tibia, as I believe it may lead to the joint being overconstrained. Backup fixation is then obtained on the tibia with a small bone staple placed to secure both grafts (**Fig. 7–42**). I once again verify that the varus instability has been eliminated, as well as the external rotation and posterolateral rotation of the tibia on the femur.

It is very important to perform an examination under anesthesia to confirm that the grafts have been securely fixed and to verify that the grafts are serving the function of preventing any increase in varus, external rotation, or posterolateral rotation of the tibia on the femur. If there is any concern that the instability has not been eliminated, consideration must be given to removal of all the securing hardware and further tightening of the graft(s).

Any concurrent cruciate ligament reconstructions that need to be performed should also be done in this same setting. Performing a staged reconstruction of the posterolateral corner structures followed by the cruciate ligament reconstruction is not recommended. The posterolateral corner reconstruction grafts would be at risk for stretching out because of the high forces placed on them in their secondary role of providing stability to the knee in the face of an ACL or a PCL tear if the cruciate ligament grafts were not also reconstructed concurrently.[46–49]

Once it has been verified that the posterolateral corner grafts have eliminated the instability of the knee after they have been fixated, attention can be turned to the closure. The anterior arm of the long head of the biceps femoris is reattached to its fibular location in an attempt to reconstitute the biceps bursa of the knee. The lateral capsular arthrotomy incision is closed with horizontal mattress 0-Vicryl sutures to hold it back into an anatomic location. The iliotibial band splitting incision is also likewise closed with a horizontal mattress 0 absorbable suture. It is essential to make sure that the common peroneal nerve is kept in sight at all times and out of the operative field. Once the fascial incisions are closed, copious irrigation is performed of the soft tissues and attention is turned to closure of the skin incision. This is done using 0 or 2–0

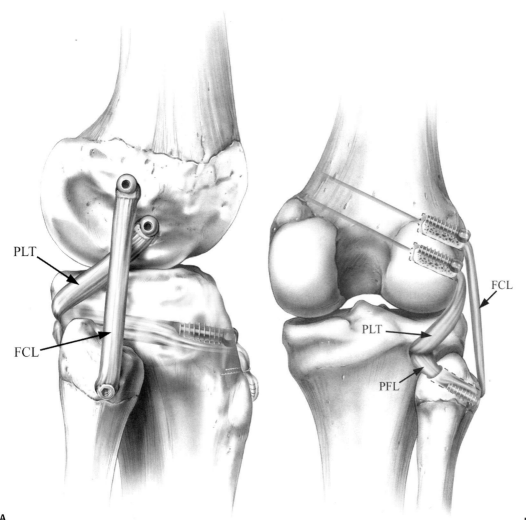

A

B

Figure 7–42   Lateral **(A)** and posterior **(B)** views of the posterolateral knee reconstruction grafts in position. FCL, fibular collateral ligament; PLT, popliteus tendon; PFL, popliteofibular ligament. (From LaPrade RF, Johansen S, Wentorf FA, Engebretsen L, Esterberg JL, Tso A. An analysis of an anatomic posterolateral knee reconstruction: an *in vitro* biomechanical study and development of a surgical technique. Am J Sports Med 2004;32:1405–1414, with permission.)

absorbable sutures, followed by a subcuticular closure of the skin with a pullout stitch. It is important to very loosely apply Steri-Strips over the lateral incision as swelling could potentially develop, which could lead to blistering of the skin due to the stretching of the skin under the Steri-Strips.

All of our patients are injected with subcutaneous Marcaine without epinephrine around the surgical incision sites to minimize postoperative pain. In a similar fashion, once the sterile dressings have been applied, patients are placed into a knee cold compression device and a knee immobilizer in full extension. Patients are kept hospitalized overnight for analgesic control and are usually discharged after seeing a physical therapist the next morning.

References

1. LaPrade RF. The medial collateral ligament complex and posterolateral aspect of the knee. In: Sports Medicine Orthopaedic Knowledge Update (OKU). Chicago: American Academy of Orthopaedic Surgeons, 1999
2. LaPrade RF, Konowalchuk BK. Popliteomeniscal fascicle tears causing symptomatic lateral compartment knee pain. Diagnosis by the Figure-4 test and treatment by open repair. Am J Sports Med 2005;33:1231–1236
3. Kannus P. Nonoperative treatment of grade II and III sprains of the lateral ligament compartment of the knee. Am J Sports Med 1989;17:83–88
4. LaPrade RF, Hamilton CD. The fibular collateral ligament–biceps femoris bursa. An anatomic study. Am J Sports Med 1997;25:439–443
5. Baker CL, Norwood LA, Hughston JC. Acute combined posterior cruciate and posterolateral instability of the knee. Am J Sports Med 1983;11:308–314
6. DeLee JC, Riley MB, Rockwood CA. Acute posterolateral rotatory instability of the knee. Am J Sports Med 1983;11:199–207
7. Krukhaug Y, Molster A, Rodt A, Strand T. Lateral ligament injuries of the knee. Knee Surg Sports Traumatol Arthrosc 1998;6:21–25
8. Terry GC, LaPrade RF. The biceps femoris muscle complex at the knee: its anatomy and injury patterns associated with acute anterolateral-anteromedial rotatory instability. Am J Sports Med 1996;24:2–8
9. LaPrade RF, Hamilton CD, Engebretsen L. Treatment of acute and chronic combined anterior cruciate ligament and posterolateral knee ligament injuries. Sports Med Arth Rev 1997;5:91–99
10. LaPrade RF, Gilbert TJ, Bollom TS, et al. The magnetic resonance imaging appearance of individual structures of the posterolateral knee. Am J Sports Med 2000;28:191–199
11. LaPrade RF. Arthroscopic evaluation of the lateral compartment of knees with grade III posterolateral knee complex injuries. Am J Sports Med 1997;25:596–602
12. LaPrade RF, Terry GC. Injuries to the posterolateral aspect of the knee: association of anatomic injury patterns with clinical instability. Am J Sports Med 1997;25:433–438
13. Jakob RP, Warner JP. Lateral and posterolateral rotatory instability of the knee. In: Jakob RP, Stäubli HU, ed. The Knee and the Cruciate Ligaments: Anatomy, Biomechanics, Clinical Aspects, Reconstruction, Complications, Rehabilitation. New York: Springer-Verlag, 1992:463–494
14. Fürst CM. Der Musculus Popliteus und Seine Sehne. Ueber ihre Entwicklung und uber Einige Damit Zusammenhangende Bildungen. Lunds Universitets Arsskrift Band 39, Lund, Germany: E. Malstroms Buchdruckerei, 1903 (German)
15. Latimer HA, Tibone JE, El Attrache NS, McMahon PJ. Reconstruction of the lateral collateral ligament of the knee with a patellar tendon allograft. Am J Sports Med 1998;26:656–662
16. Veltri DM, Warren RF. Operative treatment of posterolateral instability of the knee. Clin Sports Med 1994;13:615–627
17. Fleming RE, Blatz DJ, McCarroll JR. Posterior problems in the knee: posterior cruciate insufficiency and the posterolateral rotatory insufficiency. Am J Sports Med 1981;9:107–113
18. Hughston JC, Jacobson KE. Chronic posterolateral instability of the knee. J Bone Joint Surg 1985;67A:351–359

19. Noyes FR, Barber-Westin SD. Surgical reconstruction to treat chronic deficiency of the posterolateral complex and cruciate ligaments of the knee joint. Am J Sports Med 1996;24:415–426

20. Trillat A. Posterolateral instability. In: Schultz KP, Krahl H, Stein WH, ed. Late Reconstruction of Injured Ligaments of the Knee. Berlin: Springer, 1978:99–105

21. Clancy WG. Repair and reconstruction of the posterior cruciate ligament. In: Chapman M, ed. Operative Orthopaedics. Philadelphia: JB Lippincott, 1988: 1651–1655

22. Clancy WG, Sutherland TB. Combined posterior cruciate ligament injuries. Clin Sports Med 1994;13:629–647

23. Fanelli GC, Giannotti BF, Edson CJ. Arthroscopically assisted combined posterior cruciate ligament/posterior lateral complex reconstruction. Arthroscopy 1996; 12:521–530

24. Wascher DC, Grauer JD, Markolf KL. Biceps tendon tenodesis for posterolateral instability of the knee. Am J Sports Med 1993;21:400–406

25. Albright JP, Brown AW. Management of chronic posterolateral rotatory instability of the knee: surgical technique for the posterolateral corner sling procedure. Instr Course Lect 1998;47:369–378

26. Bousquet G, Charmion L, Passot JO, et al. Stabilisation du condyle externe du genou dans les laxites anterieures chroniques. Rev Chir Orthop 1986;72: 427–434

27. Ivey FM, Blazina ME, Fox JM, et al. Intraarticular substitution for anterior cruciate insufficiency: a clinical comparison between patellar tendon and meniscus. Am J Sports Med 1980;8:405–410

28. Arnoczky SP. Anatomy of the anterior cruciate ligament. Clin Orthop Rel Res 1983;172:19–25

29. Dye SF, Cannon WD. Anatomy and biomechanics of the anterior cruciate ligament. Clin Sports Med 1988;17:715–725

30. Acker JH, Drez D. Analysis of isometric placement of grafts in anterior cruciate ligament reconstruction procedures. Am J Knee Surg 1989;2:65–70

31. Morgan CD, Kalman VR, Grawl DM. Definitive landmarks for reproducible tibial tunnel placement in anterior cruciate ligament reconstruction. Arthroscopy 1995;11:275–288

32. Fu FH, Schulte KR. Anterior cruciate ligament surgery 1996: state of the art? Clin Orthop Rel Res 1996;325:19–24

33. Hutchinson MR, Bae TS. Reproducibility of anatomic tibial landmarks for anterior cruciate ligament reconstructions. Am J Sports Med 2001;29:777–780

34. Harner CD, Xerogeanes JW, Livesay GA, et al. The human posterior cruciate ligament complex: an interdisciplinary study. Ligament morphology and biomechanical study. Am J Sports Med 1995;23:736–745

35. Noyes FR, Barber-Westin SD. Surgical reconstruction of severe chronic posterolateral complex injuries of the knee using allograft tissues. Am J Sports Med 1995;23:2–12

36. LaPrade RF, Ly TV, Wentorf FA, Engebretsen L. The posterolateral attachments of the knee: a qualitative and quantitative morphologic analysis of the fibular collateral ligament, popliteus tendon, popliteofibular collateral ligament, and lateral gastrocnemius tendon. Am J Sports Med 2003;31:854–860

37. LaPrade RF. Posterolateral knee reconstruction. American Academy of Orthopaedic Surgeons, Surgical Procedures Section in Orthopaedic Knowledge Online (OKO), www5.aaos.org/oko/login.cfm, February 20, 2003

38. LaPrade RF, Johansen S, Wentorf FA, Engebretsen L, Esterberg JL, Tso A. An analysis of an anatomic posterolateral knee reconstruction: an *in vitro* biomechanical study and development of a surgical technique. Am J Sports Med 2004;32:1405–1414

39. Noyes FR, Barber-Westin SD, Hewitt TE. High tibial osteotomy and ligament reconstruction for varus angulated anterior cruciate ligament deficient knees. Am J Sports Med 2000;28:282–296

40. Gollehon DL, Torzilli PA, Warren RF. The role of the posterolateral and cruciate ligaments in the stability of the human knee: a biomechanical study. J Bone Joint Surg 1987;69A:233–242

41. Grood ES, Stowers SF, Noyes FR. Limits of movement in the human knee. Effect of sectioning the posterior cruciate ligament and posterolateral structures. J Bone Joint Surg 1988;70A:88–97

42. Veltri DM, Deng X-H, Torzilli PA, Warren RF, Maynard MJ. The role of the cruciate and posterolateral ligaments in stability of the knee. Am J Sports Med 1995;23:436–443

43. Veltri DM, Deng X-H, Torzilli PA, Maynard MJ, Warren RF. The role of the popliteofibular ligament in stability of the human knee: a biomechanical study. Am J Sports Med 1996;24:19–27

44. LaPrade RF. The anatomy of the deep infrapatellar bursa of the knee. Am J Sports Med 1998;26:129–132

45. Last RJ. The popliteus muscle and the lateral meniscus: with a note on the attachment of the medial meniscus. J Bone Joint Surg 1950;32B:93–99

46. Kanamori A, Sakane M, Zeminski J, Rudy TW, Woo SW. *In-situ* force in the medial and lateral structures of intact and ACL-deficient knees. J Orthop Sci 2000;5:567–571

47. Harner CD, Vogrin TM, Höher J, Ma BC, Woo SL-Y. Biomechanical analysis of a posterior cruciate ligament reconstruction: deficiency of the posterolateral structures as a cause of graft failure. Am J Sports Med 2000;28:32–39

48. LaPrade RF, Resig S, Wentorf FA, Lewis JL. The effects of grade III posterolateral knee complex injuries on anterior cruciate ligament graft force. Am J Sports Med 1999;27:469–475

49. LaPrade RF, Muench C, Wentorf FA, et al. The effect of injury to the posterolateral structures of the knee on force in a posterior cruciate ligament graft: a biomechanical study. Am J Sports Med 2002;30:233–238

8

Rehabilitation of Posterolateral Corner Knee Injuries and Related Surgeries

The rehabilitation principles for the treatment of posterolateral corner knee injuries differ for isolated versus combined posterolateral corner injuries and for acute versus chronic posterolateral knee injuries. The treatment of these injuries is continually evolving. In my training, I was told by the late Dr. Jack Hughston that all patients need to be treated in a long leg cast with a pelvic band around their waist, as well as a strut at the base of their foot to prevent external rotation, for a minimum of 4 to 6 weeks after any type of primary repair or reconstructive procedure, or there would be a very high risk of these repairs stretching out over time (**Fig. 8–1**).

Although my early treatment protocols utilized the information that I had synthesized from my sports medicine fellowship at the Hughston Clinic, I realized that it was important to look at the surgical reconstructive outcomes from other surgeries around the knee that had evolved over time. I found that the treatment of anterior cruciate and medial collateral ligament injuries had also evolved from placing patients in a cast for a period of time to prescribing accelerated rehabilitation. With this in mind, I sought to develop a more joint-friendly and patient-friendly rehabilitation protocol to treat these complicated knee injuries. I was very fortunate in that I had a high volume of injuries to treat in all of these categories, which allowed me to glean information from various patients and their outcomes to determine a proper and safe rehabilitation protocol to follow. This chapter reviews these postoperative rehabilitation protocols for the treatment of various posterolateral corner injuries.

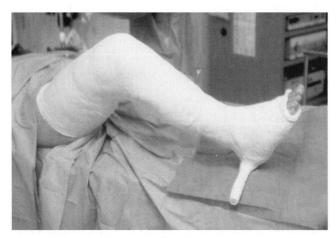

Figure 8–1.   A right knee treated in a long leg cast with a dowel rod to prevent external rotation at the foot.

◆ Isolated Acute Posterolateral Corner Injuries

The treatment of isolated acute posterolateral corner injuries depends on the amount of instability and the need for surgical intervention. For those patients who are found to have grade 1 or 2 posterolateral corner injuries, the current recommended treatment is to proceed with a nonoperative protocol.[1] These patients are treated in full knee extension, in a knee immobilizer, for a period of 2 to 3 weeks to allow for healing of the injured tissues. After this time period, they are then allowed to work on a gentle, progressive range-of-motion program as tolerated and to increase their functional activities as tolerated. During the time that they are immobilized in full extension, they are allowed to toe-touch weight bear with the use of crutches, as well as to perform quadriceps setting exercises and straight leg raises in the immobilizer only, several times daily. It is recommended that patients work on a minimum of three sets of 10 repetitions of these individual exercises daily in the immobilizer to prevent the quadriceps muscles from shutting down, which would lead to the development of quadriceps inhibition and joint effusions.

As I have noted previously, the results of nonoperative treatment of grade 3 posterolateral corner injuries is fairly dismal.[1,2] Although it is recognized that only a small number of patients need nonoperative treatment initially due to skin abrasions, open lacerations, infections, skin degloving type injuries, or other local or systemic issues, the vast majority of acute posterolateral corner injuries can be surgically repaired or reconstructed within the initial 2 weeks after injury.

◆ Acute Posterolateral Corner Surgical Rehabilitation

The main goal of any acute reconstructive procedure of the posterolateral corner of the knee is an anatomic repair that allows patients to initiate an early range-of-motion program. Ideally, I try to have them obtain full extension and a minimum of 90 degrees of knee flexion during the initial 2 to 3 weeks postoperatively. The tissues of patients who cannot be operated on within the first 2 to 3 weeks usually cannot be repaired without significant tension due to tissue retraction or an intra-substance necrosis of the tissues that does not hold sutures well. In these patients, we determine at the time of the surgical procedure what safe range of motion will be acceptable postoperatively. We then place the patient postoperatively into a hinged knee brace that is locked into this set range of motion.[3] Patients are then allowed to work within this range of motion for the initial 2 to 3 weeks after their surgical repair, or acute reconstructive procedure, and after that time are allowed to increase their range of motion as tolerated.

Overall, patients who undergo an acute posterolateral corner repair or reconstruction procedure are not allowed to bear weight on their operative extremity for a minimum of 6 weeks postoperatively. In addition, due to the potential deleterious effects of hamstring contraction on the posterolateral knee repair, they are not allowed to do any isolated open chain hamstring exercises for the initial 4 months postoperatively. It is recognized that the recommendation for avoidance of hamstring exercises is primarily based on anecdotal information that has been handed down from surgeon to surgeon over time, but avoidance of these hamstring exercises is fairly universal across most major centers that treat these injuries, and there appears to be no long-term deleterious effects of avoidance of these exercises in the initial 4 months after surgery. In addition, a recent study by Markolf et al[4] has demonstrated that quadriceps loads do increase the forces on the posterior cruciate ligament at knee flexion angles greater than 30 degrees. In light of this, I would recommend that these exercises continue to be avoided in the initial 4 months after an acute repair or reconstruction to avoid any stretching out of the operative procedure from the hamstrings pulling against the surgical repair or reconstruction.

From 2 weeks to 6 weeks postoperatively, patients are allowed to work on regaining a full range of motion of their knee. It is important that they not excessively stress their repair by trying to regain a full range of motion during this time, but it is also important to make sure that patients do not have any problems with arthrofibrosis. I have found that arthrofibrosis is a much less frequent occurrence among posterolateral corner injuries than among medial-side knee injuries. For this reason, if there is any doubt about whether sutures can hold structures after a primary repair, then one runs a small risk of having knee stiffness develop if range of motion is not initiated until 2 to 3 weeks postoperatively, unless there is a concurrent medial-side knee injury that has been addressed surgically.

During the time that patients are non–weight-bearing but allowed to work on range of motion, they work on straight leg raises and quadriceps setting exercises in an immobilizer in full extension several times daily **(Fig. 8–2)**. They are also allowed to remove their knee immobilizer to work on regaining their knee range of motion. They should not work extremely aggressively on regaining their range of motion, as this could cause stretching out of their surgical repair or reconstructive procedure during this initial healing phase after surgery.

At 6 weeks postoperatively, patients are allowed to slowly and progressively increase their weight bearing as tolerated and they may wean themselves off of crutches when they can walk without a limp. This usually takes 1 to 2 weeks after

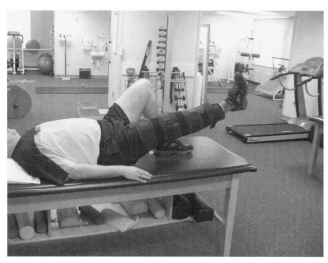

Figure 8–2   A patient performing a straight leg raise in a knee immobilizer in full extension.

they are allowed to progressively increase the weight bearing on the operative extremity. I have found that those patients who can increase their weight bearing to the point where they can wean themselves off of crutches within a couple of days postoperatively have been cheating on their weight-bearing protocol rather than keeping the operative extremity non–weight-bearing during the required time frame. Once patients are allowed to increase their weight bearing with the use of crutches, they are also allowed to work out on an exercise bike **(Fig. 8–3)**. In general, we limit patients' use of the bike to approximately 5 minutes for the first week with no resistance, and then slowly progressively increase the resistance and time on the cycling exercise over the course of the next several weeks. The main goal of the biking program for the first week should be primarily to work on regaining a full fluid

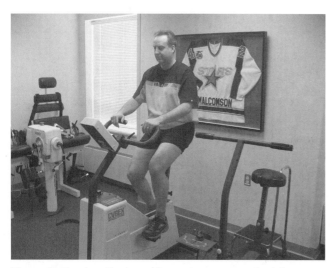

Figure 8–3   A patient working out on an exercise bike.

range of motion of the operative knee rather than working on any significant quadriceps strengthening.

In addition to the quadriceps strengthening that is regained through the use of the exercise bike, patients are also allowed to perform leg presses. In general, we allow them to utilize one quarter of their total body weight for the use of the leg press but not to flex their knee more than 70 degrees because of the cam effect of the posterior aspect of the femoral condyles on the posterior aspect of the knee. It is believed that this effect may increase the stress on the healing repair or reconstructive procedure. Frequent repetitions using the leg press within these weight limits are performed, with the nonoperative, uninjured extremity serving to back up the operative knee to make sure that excessive stress is not placed on the operative knee if it becomes fatigued while performing these exercises.

In addition to the use of the physiotherapy regimens of biking and leg presses, patients are also allowed at this time to increase their walking, as tolerated, and to swim freestyle usually using a kickboard. Patients are not allowed to perform the breaststroke or butterfly stroke yet, or to perform flip turns, to make sure that they are not putting any extra stress on their operative knee.

Patients generally follow this same conservative rehabilitation program during the initial 3 months postoperatively. They are being regularly followed to make sure that they are not having any increase in varus laxity or posterolateral rotation during the rehabilitation process. In general, most patients who follow this process have a tighter knee to varus stressing and posterolateral rotation at 3 months postoperatively than is seen in the contralateral normal knee. I allow them to return to a more aggressive rehabilitation program at 3 months, including jogging, more aggressive cycling, and increasing the weight on their leg presses. For the jogging program, patients are allowed to jog between 400 and 800 m on the first day and then they should primarily work on a walking program. If they do not notice any significant increase in pain or swelling of their knee after this initial trial, they may increase the total distance that they jog by 400 m a day until they reach a distance of 3 km, at which point they should work on a steady maintenance program of running at this distance until their knee feels more normal. They may then progressively increase their running distance up to a total of 5 km/day at 4 months postoperatively. In addition, at this time they may work up to 30 minutes/day on an exercise bike or elliptical trainer with increasing resistance as tolerated. I generally tell my younger patients that they should work as hard on the bike as they can tolerate, to the point that when they stop their legs should feel drained, but they should not feel excessively lightheaded. For those older patients or patients with a history of cardiac disease, it is recommended that they consult with their primary care physician or cardiologist prior to working on this aggressive rehabilitation program. In addition, during this period, they are allowed to work on leg presses to a maximum of 70 degrees of knee flexion, with the total weight increased as tolerated. In patients who exhibit some mild increase in laxity on their exam, a medial compartment unloader brace is used to provide backup stability to the posterolateral surgical procedure.

At 4 months postoperatively, after an acute posterolateral corner repair or reconstructive procedure, patients are evaluated to determine their overall knee stability and their functional levels. If they are still noted to have a stable and tight knee at this time, which the majority of these patients will have, they are then allowed to increase their activities as tolerated. To date, I have had more than 10 varsity intercollegiate football, basketball, track, and ice hockey athletes return to full competition at 4 months postoperatively with no long-term sequelae. All of them have noted that their knees had normal stability, and there has been no incidence of reinjury of their knees. Thus I feel that it is reasonable to allow these athletes to be treated in this rehabilitation program without the need for casting in the initial 3 to 6 weeks postoperatively.

One rehabilitation program cannot be used for all patients. In patients in the semiacute phase after injury, which is usually 4 to 6 weeks after injury, before they become chronic, there is still a chance of obtaining a primary repair as part of the operative treatment. However, the tissues are usually more significantly retracted, and suture repairs of the posterolateral structures are much more difficult. In the small subgroup of patients who may be treated, it may be appropriate to place them in a cast postoperatively for 2 to 3 weeks to make sure that they have interval healing of their primary repair technique and that they do not stretch out. I progress with their rehabilitation much more slowly than in those patients who can be treated more acutely and obtain a near-normal "safe zone" of knee range of motion after a primary repair of the torn posterolateral structures.

◆ Treatment of Acute, Combined Posterolateral Corner and Other Knee Ligament Injuries

Acute, combined posterolateral corner knee injuries usually occur with a combined anterior cruciate or posterior cruciate ligament injury. In most other patients, there is a knee dislocation that usually needs to be treated postoperatively based on the individual findings at the time of surgery rather than on a cookbook type of generic rehabilitation protocol. In general, the treatment of a combined posterolateral corner and cruciate ligament surgery is guided during the initial 6 weeks postoperatively by the posterolateral corner injury.

In acute anterior cruciate ligament and posterolateral corner knee injuries, it is desirable to allow patients to obtain full knee extension immediately after the surgical procedure. Of course, there are some instances where the posterolateral corner repair may limit the amount of knee extension that can be obtained. Once again, the surgeon can determine the safe range of motion that can be achieved intraoperatively for this combined knee ligament injury complex, without undue tension on the posterolateral corner repair procedure. It is generally desirable to obtain a range of motion of between 0 and 90 degrees within the first 2 to 4 weeks postoperatively after these combined ligament surgeries. During this time, patients are kept non–weight-bearing to prevent any increased stress on the posterolateral corner surgery. Patients are encouraged to perform quadriceps setting exercises and straight leg raises only in their immobilizers four to five times daily during this 6-week period.

After the initial 6 weeks postoperatively, patients are then allowed to progressively increase their weight bearing as tolerated and they may wean off crutches when they can walk without a limp. It is at this time that we treat these patients' as "day 1" isolated anterior cruciate ligament reconstructive knees and rehabilitate them accordingly. They are allowed to wean themselves off crutches when they can walk without a limp and to slowly increase their resistive exercises based on their overall strength and endurance. The use of an exercise bike, a general walking program, and leg presses to a maximum of 70 degrees of knee flexion is encouraged in the initial 6 to 12 weeks postoperatively for these combined ligament injuries. At 3 months postoperatively, they are allowed to increase their strengthening and to jog, based on their overall operative limb strength and the stability of their posterolateral knee repair. In general, patients take 2 to 3 months longer to recover from an acute combined anterior cruciate ligament and posterolateral corner repair surgical procedure than from an isolated anterior cruciate ligament reconstructive procedure.

◆ Treatment Protocols for Chronic Posterolateral Corner Knee Injuries

Postoperative Rehabilitation for the Posterolateral Corner Reconstruction Procedure

The posterolateral corner reconstructive procedure reconstructs the fibular collateral ligament, popliteus tendon, and popliteofibular ligament. These structures are important functionally to prevent abnormal varus opening, external rotation, and posterolateral rotation of the injured knee.[5-10] For this reason, it is important during the early postoperative rehabilitation period (6 to 8 weeks) that extra stress is not placed on these grafts by knee motions that could cause the grafts to stretch out. The grafts may not yet have healed in their bony tunnels. It is also important to make sure that the patient has appropriate muscle strength to prevent abnormal motion of their knee. It is well recognized that the function of knee ligaments is not to provide stability of the knee except in excessive amounts of knee motion. In general, patients should have strong musculature around the knee and have the muscles, rather than the knee ligaments, hold the knee together during the majority of their activities of daily living. If patients need to have the reconstruction knee ligament grafts hold their knee together during the initial few weeks to months after a surgical procedure, before their muscles are strong enough to hold their knee together, there is a very high risk that the reconstructive grafts may stretch out over time. The analogy that I describe to patients is taffy stretching out once it is pulled, or a metal coat hanger being bent back and forth and slowly breaking; similarly, these grafts suffer fatigue with these particular motions. The overall rehabilitation program that we utilize for our posterolateral corner reconstructions serves as a general guideline to patients who undergo this procedure (**Table 8–1**). This rehabilitation program may need to be modified for each patient's circumstances.

Table 8–1   Postoperative Rehabilitation Protocol for the Posterolateral Knee Reconstruction Procedure

General Overview

The posterolateral corner knee reconstruction reconstructs the popliteus tendon, the popliteofibular ligament, and fibular collateral ligament. These structures function to prevent abnormal varus opening, external rotation, and posterolateral rotation of the injured knee. Thus it is important during the early postoperative period that extra stress not be placed on these grafts with these motions so as not to cause them to stretch out until they have healed in their bone tunnels and the patient has appropriate muscle strength to prevent abnormal motion of their knee. This rehabilitation program serves as a general guideline for patients who undergo this reconstruction, but it should be individualized, especially if there is other concurrent knee ligament surgery.

Early Postoperative Modifying Factors

1. Remain in the knee immobilizer at all times other than working on knee motion or performing quadriceps exercises.
2. Remain non–weight-bearing through the end of week 6.
3. Avoid tibial external rotation (avoid external rotation of the foot/ankle, especially when sitting).
4. Avoid hamstring exercises for 4 months postoperatively.

Postop Week 1 to 2

1. Continue elevating the knee to minimize swelling.
2. Start doing quadriceps sets and straight leg raises (which should only be performed in the immobilizer). Quadriceps sets are performed hourly to tolerance, and straight leg raises in the immobilizer are performed four to five times daily.
3. Work on gentle range-of-motion (ROM) exercises four times daily outside of the immobilizer. Strive to achieve a minimum of 90 degrees of knee flexion by postoperative day 14.

Postop Weeks 3 to 6

1. Work on further quadriceps strengthening exercises as well as increasing knee ROM.
2. Continue doing quadriceps sets and straight leg raises in the knee immobilizer as the main form of exercise. Quadriceps sets should be performed in sets of 10 to 30 repetitions, five to six times daily. Straight leg raises should be performed with 10 to 12 repetitions, four times daily.
3. Work on maintenance of full knee extension several times daily. Also work on increasing knee flexion outside of the knee immobilizer five to six times daily to 90 degrees or greater.

Postop Weeks 7 to 12

1. Initiate weight bearing and low-impact closed chain exercises. Use crutches until one can walk without a limp.
2. Do quadriceps sets with 10 to 30 repetitions performed five to six times daily, and straight leg raises with 10 to 30 repetitions, performed five to six times daily.
3. Start using an exercise bike once 105 to 110 degrees of knee flexion is achieved. Work on fluid motion rather than on an increase in strength. Start out with a total of 5 minutes on the exercise bike every other day. Increase time on the bike up to 20 minutes daily based on knee response to this activity. If there is evidence of soreness or effusions developing, back off of the total minutes and days utilizing the bike.

Table 8–1 (*Continued*)

Postop Weeks 13 to 16

Goals:

1. Full knee range of motion; see surgeon if extension deficit >5 degrees or flexion <110 degrees
2. Normal gait pattern
3. Increase in functional strengthening program

Exercise Program:

1. Continue with previous exercises, daily or every other day as tolerated.
2. Weight room activities:
   a. Leg press machine: start off with 20 kg (45 lb) and perform to fatigue; knee flexion is allowed to maximum of 70 degrees.
   b. Squat rack/squat machine: half squats (not past 70 degrees of knee flexion) at half body weight, 10 repetitions; progress to full body weight as tolerated.
   c. Continue biking and/or swimming program on a daily basis. No whipkicks or flip turns allowed.

Postop Months 4 to 6

Goals:

1. Improve quadriceps strength/function
2. Increase endurance
3. Improve coordination/proprioception

Exercise Program:

1. Walking program: 20 to 30 minutes daily with medium to brisk pace. Add 5 minutes per week.
2. Biking: Increase the resistance as tolerated. Perform three to five times/week at 20 minutes per session. Thighs/legs should feel drained once off the bike.
3. Step-ups: Put foot of operative knee on step and step up on the step. Repeat with an increase in repetitions up to 100 step-ups per day. Attempt to take twice as long to step-down from the step as one takes to step-up.

Postop Months 7 and Later:

1. Continue on maintenance exercise program three to five times/week.
2. No competition or pivot sports until cleared by surgeon.
3. Strive to achieve maximum strength of the operation extremity. Even well placed and functioning grafts could stretch out over time if one relies on the grafts to make the knee stable rather than having appropriately strengthened muscles provide stability to the knee.

The main modifying factor that should occur during the initial portion of the rehabilitation program is that the patient remains in the knee immobilizer at all times other than when he or she is working on knee motion or performing quadriceps exercises. Patients should not come out of the immobilizer until they can perform a straight leg raise without a sag. In addition, patients should remain non–weight-bearing through the end of week 6 after this reconstructive procedure. It is also important to emphasize to patients that they should avoid external rotation of their foot and ankle, especially when they are sitting for periods of time, so as not to potentially stretch out their posterolateral corner reconstruction. Both Dr. Jack Hughston and Dr. Glenn Terry of the Hughston Clinic emphasized the importance of avoiding this situation during the early healing phases postoperatively. Similarly to the rehabilitation principles for an acute repair or reconstruction of posterolateral knee injuries, it is also recommended that progressive hamstring strengthening exercises be avoided during

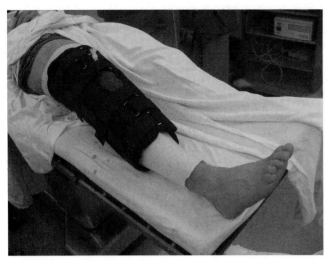

Figure 8–4   A patient in a Cryocuff and knee immobilizer in full extension postoperatively.

the initial 4 months postoperatively to avoid extra posterior and posterolateral rotatory stresses being applied to the healing reconstruction tissues.

For the initial 1 to 3 days postoperatively, patients should elevate their knee above the level of their heart to minimize postoperative swelling. An ice pack or commercial cold compression device should also be utilized to help in pain control and to minimize swelling of the operative extremity (**Fig. 8–4**). In terms of strengthening exercises, patients should initiate the use of quadriceps sets and straight leg raises, which should only be performed in their immobilizer. Quadriceps sets, in which patients maximally fire their quadriceps musculature (which is described to them as if they are going to perform a straight leg raise without actually lifting the leg off the table), are performed hourly as tolerated, whereas straight leg raises in the immobilizer only are performed four to five times daily. Early initiation of these quadriceps exercises is very important to help minimize postoperative quadriceps atrophy and the resultant knee effusions that can subsequently develop. Patients who perform these exercises on a fairly regular basis recover much more quickly, once they are allowed to initiate a range of motion and weight-bearing program, than do those patients who do not follow this rehabilitation program.

In general, patients are allowed to remove their knee immobilizer to work on gentle range-of-motion exercises four times daily. We keep most patients in full knee extension for the first 2 weeks postoperatively. Overall, the risk of arthrofibrosis with posterolateral knee injuries appears to be very low, and I have seen few problems with keeping the patients in full knee extension for 2 weeks. Between weeks 2 and 4, we ask that patients strive to achieve a minimum of 90 degrees of knee flexion. The use of a continuous passive motion machine may be indicated in some of these patients, but I have found that it rarely needs to be used postoperatively for a posterolateral corner reconstruction procedure. Most of the time it is used for acute knee dislocations rather than for combined chronic knee ligament reconstructions.

From 2 to 6 weeks postoperatively, patients work on maintaining their quadriceps strength through exercising, as well as increasing their knee range of motion. They continue to ambulate with the use of crutches with no weight bearing on their operative extremity. Quadriceps sets and straight leg raises in the knee immobilizer will continue to be the main form of exercise during this part of the rehabilitation cycle. Quadriceps sets should be performed in sets of 10 to 30 repetitions five to six times a day. Straight leg raises should be performed with 10 to 12 repetitions at least four times a day. Patients should also work on maintenance of full knee extension several times daily and on increasing the amount of knee flexion. For patients who are having problems regaining their full range of motion in flexion, a continuous passive motion machine may be indicated.

Quadriceps sets and straight leg raises are also the main forms of rehabilitation exercises in the initial 1 to 2 weeks postoperatively. If patients can perform a straight leg raise without any knee flexion sag, that is, the knee can be held out perfectly straight in extension, they are allowed to initiate quadriceps sets and straight leg raising exercises outside the knee immobilizer. Otherwise, they should continue to do these exercises in the knee immobilizer only, with 30 sets of quadriceps setting exercises, five to six times daily, and 10 to 12 straight leg raises in full extension, a minimum of five to six times daily.

Starting at 6 weeks postoperatively, patients are allowed to initiate weight bearing and low-impact, closed chain quadriceps strengthening exercises. Patients should not engage in excessive activities that could stretch out the healing reconstruction grafts. Although patients are allowed to initiate weight bearing, they should continue to use crutches until they can walk without a limp. This is to make sure that they do not put excessive stress on their reconstruction grafts until they have appropriate muscle strength to protect them. They should also avoid any significant activities until they maximize their strength gains. In addition, patients should use an exercise bike and swimming, similarly to the acute repair or reconstructive rehabilitation program that has been outlined previously. Patients who swim should not do breaststroke or a whip-kick type of stroke with their legs, as it could cause stretching out of the posterolateral corner grafts in the early healing phases.

Patients should continue to perform quadriceps setting exercises and straight leg raises during this time. Quadriceps sets with between 10 and 30 repetitions should be performed five to six times daily. Straight leg raises with similar repetitions should be performed also five to six times daily concurrently with the quadriceps setting exercises. In addition, patients should be encouraged to use an exercise bike once they achieve between 105 and 110 degrees of knee flexion. The initial goal of using the exercise bike is to work on fluid, unrestricted knee motion rather than trying to increase the overall strength of their lower extremity. They should start off with a total of 5 minutes on the exercise bike every other day. They may then increase their time on the bike up to 20 minutes daily and their overall resistance based on how their knee responds. If there is any evidence of significant soreness or effusions developing, the patient should reduce either the cycling time or the resistance.

Starting at 6 weeks postoperatively, patients are allowed to utilize a leg press machine. They should not excessively flex or place excessive stress on their knee when performing these exercises. We usually recommend that patients flex to a maximum of 70 degrees of knee flexion so as not to place extra stress or to cause posterior translation of the knee, as well as to start off with

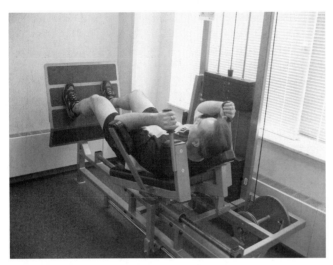

Figure 8–5   A patient performing leg presses to a maximum of 70 degrees of knee flexion.

20 kg (45 lb) on the leg press machine and to perform that exercise to fatigue **(Fig. 8–5)**. It is recommended that while patients are doing the leg presses that they use their contralateral leg to help with supporting the operative limb. Patients may also perform standing half-squats, not past 70 degrees of knee flexion, several times daily. They can perform them against a railing or a door-knob for support.

Over the period of 4 to 6 months postoperatively, the main goals of our posterolateral corner reconstruction rehabilitation program are to improve quadriceps strength and function, to increase endurance, and to improve coordination and proprioception. The exercise program during this time consists of walking 20 to 30 minutes daily, with a medium to brisk ambulation pace, adding 5 minutes per week to this protocol. In addition, the use of an exercise bike should be increased as tolerated. Three to five times per week, patients should work at 20 minutes per session to try to increase their overall quadriceps strength. Patients' thighs or legs should feel drained once they get off the bike, but they should not feel light-headed. In addition to these exercises, patients are allowed to perform step-up exercises: they put the foot of the operative knee on a step and step up on the step. This is repeated with an increase in the repetitions until they are doing 100 step-ups a day. The patient should take twice as long in stepping down as in stepping up, so as to try to gain the maximum amount of increased strength on the operative extremity.

After 6 months, patients should continue to work on a regular maintenance exercise program similar to the one noted above until they are at full strength. Patients are not allowed to participate in competitive or pivot shift type sports, such as basketball or soccer, until they have been specifically cleared by the surgeon. Patients should strive to achieve maximum strength of the operative extremity prior to returning to full functional activities. Even well-placed and well-functioning grafts can stretch out over time if one relies solely on them to make the knee stable, rather than having appropriately strengthened muscles provide stability. Thus patients who have these complex reconstructive surgeries should participate in a regular exercise program to maximize their surgical outcome.

Rehabilitation After a Proximal Tibial Opening Wedge Osteotomy

It is not uncommon in chronic posterolateral corner injuries for surgeons to perform a realignment osteotomy to correct a patient's out of varus alignment prior to proceeding with a reconstructive soft tissue procedure for the posterolateral corner of the knee. Although the rehabilitation protocol is very similar to that followed for patients who have a similar osteotomy for the treatment of osteoarthritis, it is not common for patients with chronic posterolateral corner injuries to have the same amount of arthritis as those patients who have the osteotomy for arthritis. In that regard, the rehabilitation program can usually be accelerated once the osteotomy heals for patients who undergo a proximal tibial opening wedge osteotomy and who have malalignment and underlying grade 3 posterolateral corner injuries.

Goals should be individualized for patients who have other concurrent surgeries or whose bone quality may not be normal (**Table 8–2**). A proximal tibial opening wedge osteotomy is a surgical fracture and it should be treated as a proximal tibial fracture in the initial postoperative period to allow bone healing. In addition, it is essential that patients avoid smoking or the use of nicotine, as it can significantly affect the rate and quality of bone healing. Range of motion is strongly encouraged in the early postoperative period to prevent arthrofibrosis, but weight bearing should be minimized until evidence of healing occurs and the patient is cleared by the surgeon.

For the initial 1 to 3 days postoperatively, the main goal is to make the patient comfortable and to verify that the quadriceps mechanism has initiated normal firing. Patients are allowed to ambulate with the use of crutches and are maintained in a non–weight-bearing status. Quadriceps setting exercises and straight leg raises are allowed in a knee immobilizer only. The immobilizer should be worn at all times, except to work on gentle, active range of motion of the knee four times a day. Aggressive attempts at flexion should not be allowed, to make sure that the patient does not have significant pain. Patients should also frequently elevate their operative knee, and we have found that the use of a cold compression device around the knee helps with pain control and to decrease swelling.

During weeks 1 through 6 postoperatively, healing of the osteotomy and incorporation of the bone graft is started. Patients are still kept on strict non–weight-bearing. Their goal between weeks 2 and 6 is to maintain and achieve a full range of motion of their operative knee. Gentle, active range-of-motion exercises outside the knee immobilizer are continued four times daily and may increase as strength allows. Patients are also encouraged to perform straight leg raises in a knee immobilizer several times daily to make sure that their quadriceps mechanism continues to fire adequately, and there is minimal quadriceps atrophy. The immobilizer should be worn throughout this time period to minimize the stress on the osteotomy and to decrease the chance of any subsidence at the surgical site or to cause a fracture of the lateral cortex of the tibia at the osteotomy.

Table 8–2   Proximal Tibial Opening Wedge Osteotomy Rehabilitation Protocol

Goals
The opening wedge osteotomy should be treated as a proximal tibial fracture (which in essence it is in a controlled situation) that must be treated very cautiously in the initial period after surgery to allow bone healing. Range of motion is encouraged in the early postoperative period to prevent scarring of the joint, but weight bearing should be minimized until evidence of healing occurs and it is cleared by the surgeon.

Postop Days 1 to 3

1. Main goal: obtain patient comfort and verify quadriceps firing.
2. Ambulation with crutches is initiated. Instruct patient in strict non–weight-bearing technique.
3. Quadriceps sets and straight leg raises are allowed in a knee immobilizer only. The immobilizer should be worn at all times except when working on gentle active knee motion.

Postop Weeks 1 to 6

1. Strict non–weight-bearing
2. Active range of motion is performed four times a day, and this may increase as strength allows.
3. Frequent straight leg raises in an immobilizer are performed to maintain quadriceps strength.

Postop Weeks 7 to 8

1. Initiation of range of motion and general quadriceps strengthening with an exercise bike
2. Minimal to no resistance should be applied on the stationary bicycle. Speed can be increased as tolerated depending on the patient's symptoms.

Postop Week 9

1. Based on radiographic evidence of healing, the patient is allowed to initiate weight bearing (usually increase at 25% of body weight per week through the next month).
2. The immobilizer may be discontinued. Weight bearing is advanced slowly and discontinued if the patient has pain.
3. Leg presses to a maximum of 40 lb are allowed. Perform three sets with a maximum of 20 repetitions, on a daily basis.

Postop Months 3 to 4

1. Based on evidence of radiographic healing, the patient is allowed to increase activities as tolerated.
2. Start out with the use of two crutches over the course of 7 to 14 days, until joint pain has subsided. Once this is achieved, patients are allowed to graduate to the use of one crutch under the contralateral arm.
3. Once patients can ambulate with full weight and no limp, they can graduate to using no crutches.
4. The exercise bike may be increased to 20 minutes daily with resistance as tolerated. Leg presses may also be increased to a maximum of half body weight.
5. Patients should also continue to work on a general strengthening program. Low-impact activities should be stressed.

Postop Months 5 to 6

1. Patients are allowed to return to full low-impact activities (swimming, exercise bike, walking) as tolerated.
2. Functional activities are stressed.

During weeks 7 and 8, further healing of the osteotomy site will occur. Patients can further stimulate the healing process by initiating range of motion and general quadriceps strengthening with the use of a stationary exercise bicycle; minimal to no resistance should be applied. The patient should start initially at a very slow speed and primarily work on obtaining a fluid, full range of motion of their operative knee. The speed can be increased as tolerated, depending on the patient's symptoms and response to use of the exercise bike. Otherwise, patients are kept strictly non–weight-bearing until 8 weeks postoperatively and until radiographs have been obtained that verify that it is safe to proceed to the next phase of the rehabilitation program.

Starting at postoperative week 9, based on radiographic evidence of healing of the osteotomy site, the patient is allowed to initiate weight bearing at 25% of body weight, increasing by 25% of body weight per week to full weight bearing over the course of the next month. The use of the immobilizer may be discontinued at this point if the patient can perform a straight leg raise without a sag. Weight bearing should be advanced slowly and should be discontinued if the patient has any pain at the joint line or at the osteotomy site. Most patients do not have pain with weight bearing at this time, and those who do may have some subsidence at the osteotomy site, so it is important to make sure that they stay on crutches until radiographs can be obtained to verify that it is safe to progress with further advancement of their rehabilitation program. In addition to the use of the exercise bike, patients are allowed to perform exercises on a leg press machine. They should perform knee flexion to a maximum of 70 degrees and may start off with 20 kg (45 lb) and perform leg presses to fatigue. The contralateral leg serves as a backup to prevent any excessive stress on the operative knee.

At 3 months postoperatively, radiographs are obtained to verify the healing of the osteotomy site. If there is good evidence of bone bridging at the osteotomy site and there is no evidence of screw bending or subsidence, patients are allowed to increase their weight bearing as tolerated and to wean themselves off of crutches when they can walk without a limp. We generally have them start off with the use of two crutches with full weight bearing over the course of 7 to 14 days until they have no pain at the joint line or at the osteotomy site. Once this is achieved, they are allowed to graduate to the use of one crutch under the contralateral arm to assist with weight bearing. They may then wean off this crutch when they can walk without a limp. The use of an exercise bike may increase to 20 minutes daily with increasing resistance as tolerated. Leg presses may also be increased to a maximum of one half body weight as tolerated, striving to perform three sets with a maximum of 20 repetitions a minimum of three times a week. Patients may also be allowed to work on a general lower extremity strengthening program. They may ambulate up to a maximum of 2 miles daily and should primarily perform low-impact exercises. Freestyle swimming is also allowed with no flip turns until appropriate strength is obtained.

At postoperative months 5 and 6, patients are allowed to return to full low-impact activities as tolerated. They should strive to obtain maximum quadriceps strength and to return to functional activities. Because these patients usually do not have any significant underlying arthritis and have the osteotomy for the reasons noted previously, it is our goal to have them return to near-normal activities and to stress their knee to see if they have any functional instability. In many of our patients, we have found that with the tightness provided by the opening wedge osteotomy (see Chapter 6), as well as the realignment into valgus, rather than varus, realignment, and less gapping of the lateral compartment at foot strike, patients find that they are not having the same amount of functional instability that they had prior to the osteotomy and they do not need a second-stage soft tissue posterolateral corner reconstruction. I ask patients to tell me if they are having functional instability and want to proceed with a soft tissue reconstruction of their posterolateral knee, rather than judge whether they need it based on the clinical examination.[11]

◆ Conclusion

Posterolateral corner knee injuries are some of the most difficult to treat surgically, and the rehabilitation protocol can be quite different from that for other knee surgeries. First, the rehabilitation program for posterolateral knee injuries requires a minimum of 6 weeks of non–weight-bearing to maximize the chance for healing. Second, if the surgeon finds the "safe zone" at the time of surgery, whereby one can work on the patient's knee range of motion, these injuries do not need to be treated postoperatively in casts or immobilized for up to 6 weeks. Third, it is generally accepted that any significant hamstring strengthening should be avoided during the first 4 months postoperatively to minimize any excessive stress on the healing posterolateral corner structures. Fourth, in combined concurrent knee ligament surgeries, it is important to individualize the rehabilitation program for these patients to maximize their outcomes. In most instances, isolated posterolateral corner surgical repairs or reconstructions can be rehabilitated, with patients returning to near normal or normal function within 6 to 9 months after surgery. In those patients who have concurrent combined reconstructions, this time frame may be 9 to 12 months.

References

1. LaPrade RF. The medial collateral ligament complex and posterolateral aspect of the knee. In: Sports Medicine Orthopaedic Knowledge Update (OKU), 2nd ed. Chicago: American Academy of Orthopaedic Surgeons, 1999
2. Kannus P. Nonoperative treatment of grade II and III sprains of the lateral ligament compartment of the knee. Am J Sports Med 1989;17:83–88
3. LaPrade RF, Hamilton CD, Engebretsen L. Treatment of acute and chronic combined anterior cruciate ligament and posterolateral knee ligament injuries. Sports Med Arth Rev 1997;5:91–99
4. Markolf KL, O'Neill G, Jackson SR, McAllister DR. Effects of applied quadriceps and hamstring muscle loads on forces in the anterior and posterior cruciate ligaments. Am J Sports Med 2004;32:1144–1149
5. Gollehon DL, Torzilli PA, Warren RF. The role of the posterolateral and cruciate ligaments in the stability of the human knee: a biomechanical study. J Bone Joint Surg 1987;69A:233–242

6. Grood ES, Noyes FR, Butler DL, Suntay WJ. Ligamentous and capsular restraints preventing straight medial and lateral laxity in intact human cadaver knees. J Bone Joint Surg 1981;63A:1257–1269

7. Grood ES, Stowers SF, Noyes FR. Limits of movement in the human knee: effect of sectioning the posterior cruciate ligament and posterolateral structures. J Bone Joint Surg 1988;70A:88–97

8. Veltri DM, Deng X-H, Torzilli PA, Warren RF, Maynard MJ. The role of the cruciate and posterolateral ligaments in stability of the knee. Am J Sports Med 1995;23:436–443

9. Veltri DM, Deng X-H, Torzilli PA, Maynard MJ, Warren RF. The role of the popliteofibular ligament in stability of the human knee: a biomechanical study. Am J Sports Med 1996;24:19–27

10. Veltri DM, Warren RF. Anatomy, biomechanics, and physical findings in posterolateral knee instability. Clin Sports Med 1994;13:599–614

11. Prodromos CC, Andriacchi TP, Galante JO. A relationship between gait and clinical changes following high tibial osteotomy. J Bone Joint Surg 1985;67A:1188–1194

9

Complications Associated with Posterolateral Knee Injuries

Although I have found that the risk of complications in the face of posterolateral knee injuries is relatively small, most of these injuries occur in combination with other ligament injuries or knee dislocations. The problems associated with these combined injuries need to be recognized when doing a posterolateral corner repair or reconstructive procedure. In an acute situation, we always try to perform the repair within the first 2 weeks after the injury, but there are circumstances that may prevent that.

◆ Risk of Infection or Wound Breakdown

In the acute, severely injured knee, it must be determined that the skin over the posterolateral corner of the knee has minimal chance of skin slough, infection, or localized skin necrosis prior to proceeding with surgery. In addition, it is important to make sure that there has not been an associated open knee dislocation with the potential for infection, or significant abrasions over the posterolateral corner of the knee, which could also increase the risk of infection. In those cases in which there is concern for a potential degloving-type injury over the posterolateral corner of the knee, it is appropriate to wait until the skin showed evidence of healing and the hematoma is resolved before attempting a posterolateral corner surgical procedure. In an open knee dislocation or a significant abrasion over the posterolateral corner of the knee, it is prudent to wait until the skin is healed and all hematologic studies show no evidence of active or residual infection present. Our standard blood laboratory workup includes a C-reactive protein level, erythrocyte sedimentation rate, and a complete blood count with differential. Any elevation of these laboratory values needs to be worked up further to make sure there is no residual infection present.

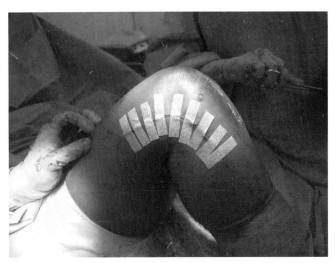

Figure 9–1   Loosely applied Steri-Strips over an acute posterolateral repair postoperatively (right knee).

In addition to the risk of skin breakdown in the acute situation, it is also important to recognize that significant postoperative swelling can develop in some of these patients. For this reason, it is important to stress that Steri-Strips placed over the surgical incision should be loosely applied **(Fig. 9–1)**. If an assistant applies Steri-Strips tightly to hold the skin edges together, postoperative swelling could result in tension and blistering of the skin, which could lead to long-term skin discoloration in this area or wound breakdown. Although a small amount of blistering might be inevitable for some of these severe injuries, it is important to be proactive and to apply the Steri-Strips very loosely rather than use them to pull the skin margins together.

In the face of chronic posterolateral knee revision reconstructions, the placement of previous skin incisions may make it difficult to perform an adequate surgical approach without crossing the skin incisions. In this circumstance, I have found it is better to incorporate the previous incision rather than to make an acute angled incision across previous incisions. In addition, it may be possible to use small horizontal incisions for an isolated fibular collateral ligament reconstruction **(Fig. 9–2)**. These issues should be discussed with the patient beforehand. Although I have not seen patients with wound breakdown in these circumstances, I have noted some mild cases of postoperative cellulitis develop in these skin flap areas, which indicates that there is a poor blood supply in the tissue flaps. These surgical wounds must be closely monitored postoperatively. In some instances, we limit the range of motion for a longer period of time, up to 2 to 3 weeks, in these patients to make sure there is no skin breakdown in the areas of a previous incision.

◆ Common Peroneal Nerve Injuries

In our series, we found that about 15% of patients with posterolateral knee injuries present with a known common peroneal nerve motor or sensory

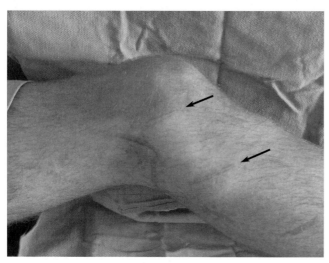

Figure 9–2   A right knee showing the location of surgical incisions (arrows) for an isolated fibular collateral ligament reconstruction after an open knee laceration that injured it.

deficit.[1] In addition, I found that a higher percentage of patients show some intrasubstance hemorrhage, bulbous swelling of the common peroneal nerve, or significant scar tissue formation along the common peroneal nerve at the time of surgery. It is important to perform a thorough physical examination of the sensory function of this nerve prior to any surgical procedures so that proper preoperative documentation of the status of the nerve is recorded that can be followed postoperatively.

In those cases in which we find a complete nerve avulsion at the time of surgery, a silk suture is tied around the ends of the nerve to identify it in the event of future nerve grafting procedures. However, in spite of seeing multiple attempts at cable grafts to reconstruct the function of the common peroneal nerve, I have not noted any patients who have had any more than a slight increase in the sensory innervation after these nerve graft procedures. I have not noted any patient to have an increase in motor function. In this regard, for patients who have evidence of a complete avulsion or tear of their common peroneal nerve at the time of surgery (**Fig. 9–3**), we recommend either a posterior tibialis tendon transfer at the same time of the initial surgery or a staged tendon transfer at 3 months postoperatively to treat their footdrop. Foot and ankle specialists are efficient in performing this tendon transfer. I have found that it significantly improves almost all patients' function so that they do not need the use of an ankle-foot orthosis and have a fairly normal gait pattern after the posterior tibialis tendon transfer.

In those acute knees that are found to have some evidence of swelling or injury to the nerve and that are noted to have some increasing motor or sensory deficits in the immediate postoperative period, we first remove the surgical dressings to try to minimize swelling around the knee. If this does not result in a resolution of the symptoms within 2 hours, we then flex the knee to 90 degrees to relieve any potential traction on the nerve. I have found that this occurs very rarely in our treated patients. The one case that I remember was a very thin young woman who

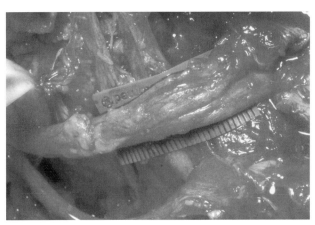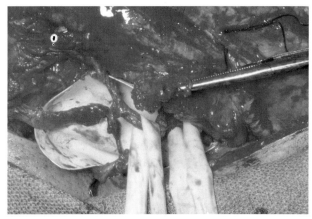

Figure 9–3   Lateral view of a right knee demonstrating both a bulbous **(A)** and avulsed (in pickups) **(B)** common peroneal nerve as part of the exposure for a severe posterolateral corner knee injury.

had a four-ligament acute knee dislocation after a snowmobile accident and developed a common peroneal nerve complete motor and sensory nerve neuropraxia overnight after all of her ligaments were reconstructed. Because I followed this protocol, she had complete return of motor and sensory function within 6 weeks postoperatively. At her 2-year follow-up, she had no residual problems.

During the surgical approach for chronic posterolateral corner injuries, it is not uncommon to find the common peroneal nerve completely encased in scar. This can be very problematic as it can add significant surgical time to the case. In addition, when the nerve is completely encased in scar, it is difficult to determine where the nerve begins and the scar tissue ends. In these circumstances, I attempt to find the common peroneal nerve either proximally, where it is just coursing under the long head of the biceps femoris, or distally, where it is just posterior to the fascia and muscle attachments of the peroneus longus muscle, at the fibular shaft. An Adson tipped hemostat is very effective in performing a common peroneal nerve neurolysis in these circumstances. It is recommended to proceed very slowly for this part of the neurolysis to obtain, at a minimum, enough decompression of the nerve such that one can gain access to the fibular head and styloid and the posterior aspect of the tibia to drill the surgical tunnels for the reconstructive procedure. I have not noted any patients who have had objective motor or sensory deficits of the common peroneal nerve after these chronic reconstruction procedures.

◆ Deep Venous Thrombosis

As in all major knee injuries, there is an increased risk for deep venous thrombosis in patients who have a posterolateral corner injury, whether it is treated in isolation or combined with other ligament injuries around the knee. Because these patients are treated with a non–weight-bearing protocol immediately after surgery for 6 weeks, they are treated prophylactically with enteric-coated aspirin, one daily, during this 6-week period. For those patients who have an allergy to aspirin, other factors that place them at a higher risk of deep venous thrombosis, or a previous history of deep venous thrombosis or pulmonary embolism (such as factor V Leiden deficiency), we commonly work with a hematologist to determine the proper postoperative anticoagulation program. In most circumstances, we start off with one of the injectable anticoagulants for the first several days to 2 weeks and then usually progress to an outpatient warfarin protocol, striving for an international normalized ratio (INR) of 1.5 to 2.0. A nurse monitors their coumadin dosage and INR levels.

If there is any doubt whether a patient has a deep venous thrombosis due to postoperative calf pain or swelling, we ask that they go to the emergency room and undergo a venous duplex ultrasound of their lower extremities to rule out a deep venous thrombosis. To my knowledge, we have not had one of these to date with our prophylactic protocol, but if one is found, the patient would be appropriately treated with anticoagulation therapy to address the deep venous thrombosis or to have it closely monitored, if it is felt by the treating hematologist to be amenable to continued observation within the patient's anticoagulation protocol.

◆ Previous Reconstructions and Retained Hardware

In addition to the concerns about previous surgical incisions for posterolateral corner reconstructions, retained hardware over the posterolateral corner of the knee can make it difficult, on occasion, to perform a surgical reconstruction. There are times when large 6.5-mm screws and washers are placed to perform a tenodesis-type procedure or a direct repair of all structures using a washer on the femur (**Fig. 9–4**). Similar hardware is sometimes placed into the fibula or even the tibia. Although we have not found the tibial hardware to be a

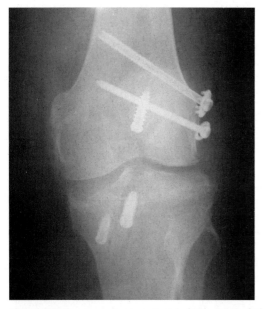

Figure 9–4 An anteroposterior (AP) view of the left knee demonstrating retained hardware with previous biceps tenodesis screws on the femur.

particular problem in the identification of the normal attachment sites of these important posterolateral structures, the hardware that is in the femur or the fibula can be problematic at times.

In evaluating the issues dealing with previous femoral hardware, it is important to find the normal bony landmarks that are present to assist in the placement of surgical reconstruction tunnels. If one can find the popliteal sulcus and the lateral epicondyle, then it is possible that some remnants of the native popliteus tendon or the fibular collateral ligament, respectively, may be found and the normal attachment sites readily identified. In those instances where the previous hardware was placed at these locations and it obliterated the normal attachment sites, one needs to rely on the measurement techniques that we outlined previously in our quantitative anatomy studies to determine the distances between the different attachment sites on the femur to best judge the correct attachment sites for these reconstructive tunnels.[2] It is especially important in these circumstances to leave the islet-tipped pins in place and to obtain all the necessary measurements to reference structures to place these tunnels in the desired anatomic attachment site positions.

Fibular head hardware can consist of either large buried suture anchors or previous screws and washers placed in for reconstructive procedures **(Fig. 9–5)**. I have not found it to be a significant problem to identify the normal attachment sites of the fibular collateral ligament and the popliteofibular ligament on the fibular head and styloid, even if previous screws and washers are placed

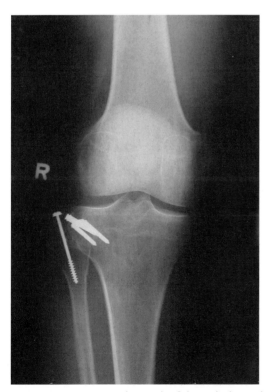

Figure 9–5   An AP radiograph of the right knee demonstrating retained fibular hardware with a screw and a washer placed in the fibular head and styloid.

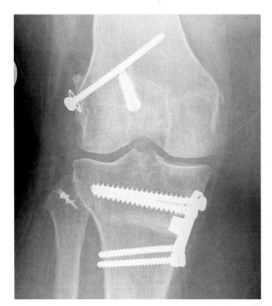

Figure 9–6 An AP view of the right knee demonstrating a retained suture anchor in the fibular head that interferes with fibular tunnel placement after a failed posterolateral surgery.

in this location. The biggest problem that I have seen is when drilling the fibular tunnel. One needs to make sure that it is drilled so that it does not break through its superior cortex, and the tunnel placement needs to be adjusted slightly if there is previous hardware that could interfere with this function. In addition, it can be very difficult to drill around large metal suture anchors that are buried in bone **(Fig. 9–6)**. What I have commonly attempted to do is to either use a very small (4 or 5 mm) reamer over the tunnel guide pin, or to ream the normal size for the tunnel and then attempt to remove the metal anchor once it is encountered. Luckily, most of the standard metal anchors can be reamed around in the process of placing these tunnels.

Retained hardware may also be present from a previous proximal tibial osteotomy. Though we do not recommend closing wedge osteotomies due to the fact that they may increase the laxity present on the lateral compartment of the knee, there are times when a well-done closing wedge osteotomy has been performed, and these staples need to be removed. These can usually be removed through the standard surgical incision over the posterolateral corner of the knee without any significant problems.

In those knees that have a previous proximal tibial opening wedge osteotomy present, it is important to remove any screws that course transversely across the tibia that may interfere with drilling the posterolateral and cruciate ligament tunnels. Removing these screws has not been found to be a problem with the standard hardware currently used for these systems **(Fig. 9–7)**.

However, in patients who had subsidence of their osteotomy to some degree and broken hardware due to this subsidence, and still have not subsided into varus alignment that would need to be corrected before any soft tissue posterolateral corner reconstruction, removal of any broken screws can be problematic **(Fig. 9–8)**. In this circumstance, it is important to make sure either

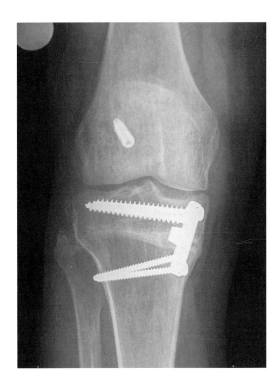

Figure 9–7 Retained hardware after a healed proximal tibial open wedge osteotomy in a patient with a chronic posterolateral knee injury; AP view of the right knee.

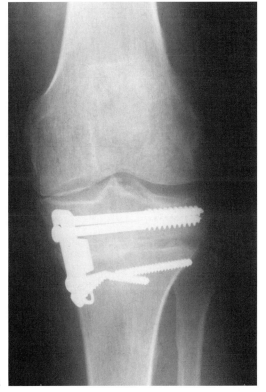

A

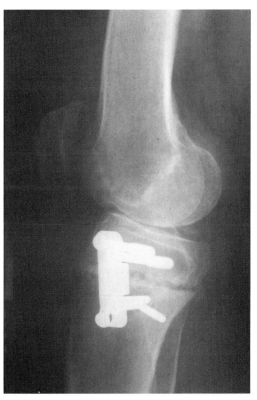

B

Figure 9–8 **(A)** AP radiograph of the right knee demonstrating broken screws after a delayed union in a proximal tibial open wedge osteotomy. **(B)** Lateral view of the left knee. Although the patient was treated for genu varus and medial compartment arthritis, broken screws after an osteotomy can interfere with reconstruction tunnel placement.

that the tunnels can be drilled around the broken screw, or that fluoroscopic imaging and the equipment to remove broken screws is available to allow for these tunnels to be placed in the proper position.

◆ Postoperative Arthrofibrosis

The risk of postoperative arthrofibrosis in acute posterolateral corner injuries depends on whether there are any other associated knee ligament injuries, especially for injuries to the medial collateral ligament complex. For acute isolated posterolateral corner knee injuries, we have found the incidence of arthrofibrosis to be rare and I have not had to bring a patient back to surgery for manipulation or debridement in this circumstance. Likewise, it is relatively rare to have arthrofibrosis develop in the face of a combined acute ACL and posterolateral corner knee injury, but I have had to bring some patients back for a manipulation and debridement because of severe scar tissue formation in this injury pattern due to the severe injury of their posterolateral structures. In these circumstances, these patients were noted to have a complete avulsion of the biceps femoris and all of the structures that attach to the fibular head, as well as the lateral capsule off the tibia. In these circumstances, we wait a minimum of 10 to 12 weeks after surgical repair prior to bringing the patients to surgery. We attempt an arthroscopic debridement of the suprapatellar pouch prior to any manipulation of the knee so as not to tear apart any of the posterolateral corner structures.

In cases in which there is an associated medial collateral ligament complex injury, usually indicating a knee dislocation with all four major ligaments of the knee torn, there is a higher risk of arthrofibrosis with operating in the acute setting. I inform patients of this risk and tell them that treatment of knee dislocations within this time frame results in a better chance of overall knee stability, and that waiting for surgical treatment until the injury becomes chronic results in a higher risk of residual laxity even if the structures are subsequently later repaired or reconstructed. I have also noted that if we do need to bring patients back for a manipulation and debridement, there appears to be no difference in the subjective and objective findings at 1 year postoperatively between these patients and other patients who have not needed a manipulation and debridement. In that regard, about 30% of our four ligament knee reconstructive surgeries do need to return to surgery for a manipulation and debridement postoperatively. In all of these patients, we strive to obtain full knee extension initially, especially to eliminate any posterior sag of the tibia on the femur that could stretch out a posterior cruciate ligament reconstruction graft or potentially a posterolateral reconstruction procedure. We have minimally had to perform an arthroscopic posterior capsular release to address extension deficits in these patients. In the majority of circumstances in which patients develop postoperative arthrofibrosis, they are able to flex only from 0 to 80 or 85 degrees by 3 months postoperatively. These patients are returned to surgery, and their suprapatellar pouch and other scar tissue encountered in the knee are debrided. Following a similar protocol as noted above, these patients are hospitalized for 2 to 3 days with an indwelling epidural catheter, and we use either a dynamic extension splint to assist with regaining full knee extension, or most commonly a continuous passive motion machine through a full range of motion to maintain the flexion gained in surgery. Our goal at the time of the manipulation and arthroscopic debridement is to obtain the same range of motion on the operative knee as on the contralateral normal knee.

In chronic posterolateral corner reconstructions, we generally attempt a program of early knee motion as part of the patients' rehabilitation protocol. The only time where I have held off on starting early range of knee motion is in patients who have combined posterior cruciate ligament reconstructions and who are found to have very osteopenic bone and if I am concerned about tibial fixation for the posterior cruciate ligament reconstruction graft. In these circumstances, I commonly keep the patient's knee out in full extension for 1 to 2 weeks to allow for early posterior cruciate ligament tibial tunnel healing to occur prior to initiation of range of motion. Once again, in these circumstances, I bring approximately one patient back to surgery per year for a debridement. Usually this debridement is of the suprapatellar pouch as the patients do not lose extension, but they sometimes lose flexion. We treat this by debridement of the suprapatellar pouch and manipulation, followed by placement of an indwelling epidural catheter and the use of a continuous passive motion machine set to a full range of motion. Patients are treated with this protocol for 2 to 3 days in the hospital. It has been found to help them to regain most of their motion deficits.

As in all cases of arthrofibrosis, the best way to treat it is to avoid it in the first place. However, there are circumstances where tissue necrosis and retraction requires patients to be kept immobile for a period of time to allow these required tissues to heal. It is usually in these patients that we see a greater need for subsequent manipulation and debridement to regain range of motion. In the future, growth factors and other treatments may minimize the chance of arthrofibrosis in these patients, but at present it is recommended to err on the side of making sure that the ligaments heal and having a small risk of stiffness, rather than to start knee motion too early and have a retearing or attenuation of the repaired structures with a more aggressive rehabilitation program.

◆ Recurrent Laxity or Instability

In patients who are felt to have significant motor weakness and who may develop residual laxity of the reconstruction grafts because they are relying on the grafts to hold their knee together, I commonly place them into a medial compartment unloader brace postoperatively to minimize any further stretching out of their grafts. I have found this to be an effective tool for providing stability to the patient's knee and to protect the reconstruction grafts. I tell patients that they should anticipate wearing this unloader brace for 1 year postoperatively, if necessary.

In patients who are found to have recurrent instability, a thorough workup must be repeated to determine the etiology of the instability. Long-leg alignment x-rays must be obtained again to verify that they are not in varus alignment; AP and lateral radiographs should be obtained to determine any medial compartment arthrosis or sagittal tibial slope alignment changes. The presence of any concurrent other ligament instability to the knee must be assessed on clinical examination.

There is an important intricate relationship between the anterior cruciate ligament and the posterolateral corner. Failure to treat either one at the time of a surgical reconstruction of the other has a high risk of either reconstruction procedure stretching out over time. There is also a reciprocal relationship between the posterior cruciate ligament and the posterolateral corner of the knee, and it is also recommended that they be reconstructed currently. In those cases in which it is recognized that there is cruciate ligament laxity that was not addressed, it should be addressed in a concurrent future reconstruction procedure. Assessment of posterolateral corner hardware placement, tunnel placement, and possibly repeat magnetic resonance (or computed tomography) imaging may be necessary to verify that these tunnels do not have significant osteolysis and are placed in the desired position. In those circumstances in which it is felt that, in retrospect, the tunnels may have been placed in a less than desired position, or in which there is sufficient tunnel osteolysis where it may be difficult to perform a revision reconstruction, it is recommended that a two-stage surgery be performed. In the first stage, a removal of hardware, debridement of scar tissue in the tunnels, and bone grafting of the tunnels are recommended. The second-stage revision reconstruction could then be performed once the knee showed evidence of healing of the bone-grafted tunnels. This would commonly be present at 6 to 9 months postoperatively.

There may also be circumstances where a patient sustains a recurrent trauma to the knee and tears the reconstruction graft due to this trauma. The same workup is recommended as described earlier, with care to make sure that the tunnels do not have osteolysis and that the reconstruction graft can be placed back in the same anatomic position (**Fig. 9–9**).

◆ Conclusions

The complications associated with the treatment of posterolateral knee injuries are similar to those associated with other knee ligament injuries. In the acute situation, it is important to assess skin integrity and potential subcutaneous

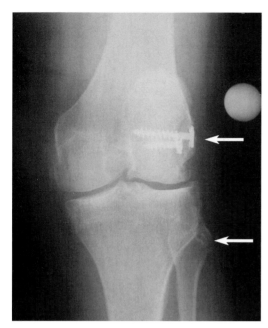

Figure 9–9   An AP radiograph of a left knee demonstrating previous reconstructive graft tunnels on the femur (and hardware) and fibula (arrows) after a failed posterolateral knee reconstruction.

hematoma and swelling, to be able to judge if there is an increased risk of infection or wound breakdown due to the damage to the subcutaneous tissues over the posterolateral corners of the knee. In addition, concurrent open lacerations or abrasions need to be properly evaluated and treated to make sure that a secondary infection does not occur.

The same principles occur to some degree for the treatment of chronic posterolateral injuries. Previous incisions need to be properly evaluated as to whether they should be incorporated or crossed perpendicular as part of the reconstructive approach. Previous hardware needs to be evaluated so that the instruments needed for hardware removal are available. The hardware's effects on the placement of reconstructive tunnels for a posterolateral corner procedure also need to be evaluated.

Postoperative management entails closely watching the patient for signs of infection, with a strong emphasis on following the rehabilitation principles and minimizing the chance of a deep venous thrombosis through prophylactic protocols. Careful monitoring of these conditions should minimize the risk of complications associated with posterolateral corner knee surgeries.

References

1. LaPrade RF, Terry GC. Injuries to the posterolateral aspect of the knee: association of anatomic injury patterns with clinical instability. Am J Sports Med 1997;25:433–438
2. LaPrade RF, Ly TV, Wentorf FA, Engebretsen L. The posterolateral attachments of the knee: a qualitative and quantitative morphology of the fibular collateral ligament, popliteus tendon, popliteofibular ligament and lateral gastrocnemius tendon. Am J Sports Med 2003;31:854–860

Index

Page numbers followed by *f* or *t* indicate figures or tables, respectively.